Physical Agents in

Physiotherapy

Principles and Practice: Volume 1

Biophysics and Therapeutic Electricity

Subin Solomen
BPT, MPT (Manipal) CRD
Professor, EMS Memorial Co-operative Hospital and Research Centre
Perinthalmanna, Kerala

Pravin Aaron
BPT, MPT (Manipal) CRD
Professor and Principal
Padmashree Institute of Physiotherapy
Bangalore, Karnataka

Peepee Publishers and Distributors (P) Ltd. ®

Physical Agents in
Physiotherapy
Principles and Practice: ***Volume 1***
Biophysics and Therapeutic Electricity

Published by
Pawaninder P. Vij and Anupam Vij

Peepee Publishers and Distributors (P) Ltd.
Head Office: 160, Shakti Vihar, Pitam Pura
Delhi-110 034 (India)

Correspondence Address:

7/31, First Floor, Ansari Road, Daryaganj
New Delhi-110002 (India)

Ph: 011-41512412, 011-23246245, 9811156083

e-mail: peepee160@yahoo.co.in

e-mail: peepee160@gmail.com

www.peepeepub.com

First Edition: **2017**
Revised Edition: 2022

ISBN: 978-81-8445-293-8

Dedicated to

My Parents, SV Solomen and Premila Solomen, My Wife Divya

And to my Children, Angelina and Jerome

– Prof Subin Solomen

Dedicated to

My Students

– Prof Pravin Aaron

Foreword

It is a matter of great pleasure and privilege to me to write this "Foreword" for the book **Physical Agents in Physiotherapy–Principles and Practice: Volume I–Biophysics and Therapeutic Electricity.**

Not many textbooks and reference books on the subject are available today that comprehensively address the subject and in this context, the present book in this format is perhaps the first one of its kind, needs to be essentially accorded its due significance. I congratulate for this commendable contribution, which has come at a time universities across the country are deciding to streamline the curriculum.

As a matter of real pride, I am very happy to note that both the authors are associated with Padmashree Institute of Physiotherapy, Bangalore and they have rightly decided to publish this work in its vicennial year.

I have gone through the contents and find that the book has been very thoughtfully developed, covering the different facets of Electrophysics and in an orderly sequence and easy to read format. The authors have indeed taken tremendous pain in preparing the book, focusing great attention to basics as well as advanced aspects and yet keeping the flow of the text simple and readable and laced with suitable examples that would help any student and teacher alike in understanding and enjoying the aspects of Biophysics and Therapeutic Electricity.

The book has 50 chapters, richly illustrated with diagrams, sketches, tables and examples providing an excellent presentation of the subject. The book undoubtedly carries the rich experience of the authors as teachers of the subject as this gets truly reflected in the depth of the information given in the book.

Dr Ashwath Narayan

MLA, Malleshwaram Constituency, Bengaluru

Managing Trustee

Padmashree Group of Institutions

Preface

The series book titled **"Physical Agents in Physiotherapy: Principles and Practice"** which is intended to cover all modalities in terms of Electrical modalities, Thermal (superficial, deep heating and Cryotherapy), Mechanical modalities (Traction and Pneumatic Compression etc.) both in terms of theoretical principles and its practical application. The series is divided into five volumes; Volume I: Biophysics and Therapeutic Electricity, Volume II: Electrophysiology, Volume III: High Frequency Currents, Actinotherapy and Acoustics, Volume IV: Superficial and Manual Modalities, Volume V: Practical Applications of Physical Agents in Physiotherapy. This series of book has been compiled and made as per the curriculum according to the draft "Model Curriculum Handbook–Physiotherapy" prepared by Allied Health Section, Ministry of Health and Family Welfare (2015–16). The syllabuses of electrotherapy in different universities in India and abroad were also taken into consideration while writing this book. The readers for this textbook series are under graduates, postgraduates, clinicians and academicians in the field of physiotherapy.

In this Volume I, it is divided into two sections; Section A: Biophysics and Section B: Therapeutic Electricity. Section A covers the Biophysics which is related to Therapeutic Currents. Section A has 25 chapters. Each topic is covered in detail with simple explanations, easy drawn pictures and its application of the physiotherapy. Electric, magnetic and thermal effect of electric current is covered in detail. Section B has 25 chapters. Initial chapters cover types of current used in physiotherapy and its effects on body, Basic nerve muscle physiology, Basics of application of currents, Structure of stimulator, Principles of applications and classification of current. Types of current detailed are Faradic current, Galvanic current, Therapeutic direct current, Iontophoresis, Sinusoidal currents, Diadynamic current, Hi-voltage Pulsed Galvanic Stimulation, Russian current, Rebox current, Micro current, TENS and IFT. A separate chapter on pain is included which covers neurobiology, mechanism, theories of pain and well detailed explanation of pain gate theories were included. Each current is discussed under definition, types, physiological effects, therapeutic effects and indications separately. Contraindications, dangers and precautions were given together in the Chapter 37. Practical application list of all currents is given in the Chapter 40. The student will gain solid foundation by going through the Biophysics. Clinicians will benefit from chapters of therapeutic electricity and practical approaches to pain gate theories. Academicians can use this textbook for teaching the students and also who wish to update their knowledge. There are around 165 figures and 30 tables in this Volume I which can be easily drawn by the students. Some of the chapters cover special points covered under heading as "Hot Spot" in the form of questions and answer. This questions and answers make the reader enthusiastic in the electrotherapy subject. These clarifications are not given in any of the similar textbooks. I hope my hard work will give noteworthy contribution to the teachers and students. Any suggestions or corrections are most welcome and can be mailed me at subins2001@rediffmail.com.

Prof. Subin Solomen

Acknowledgements

First and foremost I would like to thank almighty God without whose blessing this book would have not been possible. I would like to thank my parents who had a belief on me and always praying for my best. I also want to thank the readers and purchasers of the first edition of this book.

It's been 11 years I am teaching the electrotherapy subject. During this period, I have been teaching students from different states of India; from south to north, from east to west and also from abroad; Nepal, Sri Lanka, Bhutan, Iran, Africa, etc. The scripts on physical agents was made because of doubts, asking explanations and enthusiasm, from my dear students: Mr Deepak Joshi, Mr Bijay, Ms Sakuna and Ms Mahima. So, at this moment I want to acknowledge them. They inspired me to write a book. I would also like to thank Ms Reema, Ms Asmita, Mrs Trupti, Ms Arpana and Ms Shaily who wrote my first written notes of Lectures on electrotherapy.

I am sincerely obliged to Prof Pravin Aaron, Principal, Padmashree Institute of Physiotherapy, who is also the second author of this book. He helped me in reviewing and correcting the manuscript of this book. It was impossible to deliver this book without him. I am indebted to my Principal, Jinson K Paul, Dr A. Mohammed, Chairman, Sri M. Adunnasir, General Manager of EMS Cooperative Hospital and Research Centre, Perinthalmanna, Kerala for providing me support for writing this book. I am indebted to TK Narayanappa, Chairman, Dr CN Ashwath Narayan, Managing Trustee, Dr Vasudeva, Director and Prof Rajesh Shenoy, Director of Padmashree Group of Institutions, Bangalore where I did my graduation and worked as lecturer to professor for their support and cooperation in writing this book.

I owe my special thanks to Mr Pawaninder Pal Vij and whole team members of Peepee Publishers and Distributors for publishing the book in a nice manner. I have taken lot of information from the books published on electrotherapy which I have mentioned in the last as "List of References". I thank all the authors written on topics of electrotherapy both published and unpublished as I have borrowed information and ideas from these books.

I owe my thanks to Ms Neena Mathew Aaron, Professor, Padmashree Institute of Physiotherapy for giving significant contribution in writing chapters on nerve muscle physiology and pain. I also especially thank my brother Prabin Solomen Electrical and Electronics engineer; Qatar for teaching me applied physics which helped me a lot in writing biophysics. I also thank my friends Jimshad and Toms for their support and cooperation towards the successful completion of the book. My thanks go to my wife Divya who was continuously encouraged and supported me in writing and completion of the book for the last ten years.

Prof. Subin Solomen

Contents

1

Structure of Atom, Ions, Element, Compound and Molecules

ATOM

An atom may be defined as the smallest particle of an element that can take part in a chemical reaction. Every solid, liquid, gas, and plasma is composed of neutral or ionized atoms. Atoms are very small; typical sizes are around 100 pm (a ten billionth of a meter, in the short scale).

Structure of an Atom

All atoms are built up from three basic types of particle; protons, neutrons and electrons. Protons carry positive charge, electrons carry negative charge and neutrons carry same mass of a proton with no charge. The protons and neutrons are held together by a very strong cohesive force to form the central nucleus of the atom. The electrons revolve around the central nucleus at a very high speed. They are held in the atom by the force of attraction exerted on them by the positively charged central nucleus. The number of protons in an atom is very important as it determines the element of which it is an atom. This is known as atomic number of the element. The protons and neutrons form practically all the mass of the atom and the number of these particles together gives the atomic weight of the element. Atoms of an element which contain different numbers of neutrons are known as isotopes of that element (same atomic number different mass number). Whereas Isobars differ in atomic number (or number of protons) but have the same mass number.

IONS

If the atom gains electrons, the number of electron exceeds that of protons and particles have a negative charge, while if electrons are lost, the number of protons is greater than that of electrons and the charge is positive. Such charged particles are called ions. The negative charged ions are called anions which move towards anode (e.g., chloride ion–Cl^-). The positively charged ions are called cations which move towards cathode (e.g., sodium–Na^+).

RADICALS

Radicals are groups of atoms which are frequently found in union with each other. Examples are the carbonate (CO_3), Sulphate (SO_4) and hydroxyl radicals (OH). The atoms of these radicals are united by shared electron bonds but do not achieve a complete outer electron shell. Thus they tend to acquire more electrons and form negative ions. They behave like the atoms of elements and can enter into formation of electrovalent or covalent compounds. For example, hydroxyl ions can form electrovalent compound like sodium hydroxide and a covalent compound like zinc hydroxide.

ELEMENTS

An element may be defined as a species of atoms having the same number of protons in their atomic nuclei. It is a basic substance which cannot be split into simpler substances. There are 118 elements that have been identified, of which the first 94 occur naturally on Earth with the remaining 24 being synthetic elements.

COMPOUND AND MOLECULE

A compound is a substance formed by the union of two or more elements. A molecule is the smallest particle of any substance, element or compound that can exist alone. All compounds are molecules but not all molecules are compounds. Molecular hydrogen (H_2), molecular oxygen (O_2) and molecular nitrogen (N_2) are not compounds because each is composed of a single element.

A compound may be either electrovalent or covalent. An electrovalent compound occurs where an atom of one element gives an electron to the atom of another element. So, the first one is a positive ion and second one is negative ion. Both of them held to each other as unlike charges attract. An example is sodium chloride (Na^+, Cl^-). A covalent compound occurs where the outer shells of the atoms of the elements share a common bonding of electrons so that each atom has a complete outer shell. An example is methane (CH_4). Carbon and hydrogen contribute electrons for the outer orbit.

2

Matter

DEFINITION

Matter may be defined as 'that which occupies space and has mass'. They are either made up of elements or compounds. Matter is anything that has *mass* and *volume* (occupies *space*). For example, a car would be said to be made of matter, as it has mass and volume (occupies space).

Difference Between Matter and Mass

'Matter' is defined as 'anything that occupies space and has mass' and 'mass' is defined as "something that represents the amount of matter in a particular space, particle or object". Matter can be seen while mass is only quantifiable. The unit of mass is kilogram while matter can be measured using different forms of units of measurement, such as, weight, mass, or volume. Mass is a conserved quantity, which means that its value is unchanging through time, within closed systems. However, matter is not conserved in such systems. Matter may disappear by conversion into energy, even inside closed systems, and it can also be created from energy, within such systems. However, because mass (like energy) can neither be created nor destroyed, the quantity of mass and the quantity of energy remain the same during a transformation of matter (which represents a certain amount of energy) into non-material (i.e., non-matter) energy. This is also true in the reverse transformation of energy into matter.

Properties of Matter

Physical properties: The measurement of mass and other characteristics that can be seen without changing how that object looks are its physical properties. When you look at oranges, you know that they are oranges because of their color, shape, and smell. Mass, color, shape, volume, and density are some physical properties. Density is an important physical property. Density is the mass of a substance per unit volume. Volume is the amount of space an object occupies.

Chemical properties: These are properties that can only be observed by changing the identity of the substance. A piece of paper burns and turns to a black substance. After the flame goes out you can no longer burn the new substance. The chemical properties have been changed.

States (Phases) of Matter

Matter exists in classical state and exotic state:

Classical State

Solid

Liquid

Gas

Exotic State

Plasma

Bose–Einstein condensates

Fermionic condensates

Quark–gluon plasma

Characteristics of solids, liquid and gas are mentioned in the Table 2.1. Description of exotic states of matter is beyond the scope of this textbook.

Table 2.1: Characteristics of matter

Solid	*Liquid*	*Gas*
Retains a fixed volume and shape	Assumes the shape of the part of the container which it occupies	Assumes the shape and volume of its container
Rigid – particles locked into place	Particles can move/slide past one another	Particles can move past one another
Not easily compressible	Not easily compressible	Compressible
Little free space between particles	Little free space between particles	Lots of free space between particles
Does not flow easily	Flows easily	Flows easily
Rigid – particles cannot move/ slide past one another	Particles can move/slide past one another	Particles can move past one another

Solid: The wood block is solid. A solid has a certain size and shape. The wood block does not change size or shape. Other examples of solids are the computer, the desk, and the floor.

Liquid: Milk is a liquid. Milk is liquid matter. Liquids can flow, be poured, and spilled. If the liquid falls it will take the shape of the floor and the floor is expansive limitless boundary (until it hits the wall).

Gas: Oxygen is a gas but you can't see it and it is invisible. Gases have no color. Gases are all around you. You can feel gas when the wind blows. The wind is moving air. Air is combination of many gases mixed together.

Changing States of Matter

All matter can move from one state to another. Molecules can move from one physical state to another and will not change their basic structure. Water (H_2O) is an example. It has the same molecular structure whether it is a gas, liquid, or solid. Although its physical state may change, its chemical state remains the same. If energy is added (like increasing the temperature) or if energy is taken away (like freezing something), you have created a physical change. To create a solid, you might have to decrease the temperature by a huge amount and then add pressure. For example, oxygen (O_2) will solidify at –361.8 degrees Fahrenheit (–218.8 degrees Celsius) at standard pressure. However, it will freeze at warmer temperatures when the pressure is increased.

Points of Change

Phase changes happen when certain points are reached. A freezing point is the measure where temperature at which a liquid turns into a solid. Other points are mentioned in the Table 2.2. There are physical effects that can change the melting point. Pressure is one of those effects. When the pressure surrounding a substance increases, the freezing point and other special points also go up. It is easier to keep things solid when they are under greater pressure. Generally, solids are denser than liquids because their molecules are closer together. The freezing process compacts the molecules into a smaller space. There are always exceptions in Science. Water is special on many levels. It has more space between its molecules when it is frozen. The molecules organize in a specific arrangement that takes up more space than when they are all in the liquid state. Because the same number of molecules takes up more space, solid water is less dense than liquid water.

Table 2.2: Points of change in matter

Term	*Phase change*
Fusion/Melting	Solid to Liquid
Freezing	Liquid to Solid
Vaporization/Boiling	Liquid to Gas
Condensation	Gas to Liquid
Sublimation	Solid to Gas
Deposition	Gas to Solid

Forces that Influences the Molecules of a Matter

Cohesive force: The force which attracts the molecules of the substances to one another.

Kinetic force: The force of movement of the molecules which is dependent on the thermal energy contained by the mass of molecules.

The solid state is characterized by a dominance of potential energy (cohesive forces) over kinetic energy (disruptive forces). As a result, the particles of solids are held in rigid three-dimensional lattices in which the particle's kinetic energy takes the form of vibrations about each lattice site.

The liquid state is which neither potential energy (cohesive forces) nor kinetic energy (disruptive forces) dominates. As a result, particles of liquids are randomly arranged but are relatively close to each other and are in constant random motion, sliding freely over each other but without enough kinetic energy to become separated. The gaseous state is characterized by a complete dominance of kinetic energy (disruptive forces) over potential energy (cohesive forces). As a result, particles move randomly, essentially independently of each other. Under ordinary pressure, the particles are separated from each other by relatively large distances, except when they collide.

As more energy is added to the solid, the kinetic energy increases, molecule movement increases, structure collapses the liquid state is reached. If still more heat is applied kinetic energy is much greater than cohesive forces that molecules fly apart to form a gas.

Properties of Matter

Adhesion and cohesion: Adhesion is the tendency of dissimilar particles or surfaces to cling to one another and cohesion refers to the tendency of similar or identical particles/surfaces to cling to one another. Liquids have cohesion and adhesion, both of which are forms of molecular attraction. Cohesion enables a liquid to resist tensile stress, while adhesion enables it to adhere to another body. Cohesion allows for surface tension, creating a 'solid-like' state upon which light (in weight) or low-density materials can be placed and capillarity results from a combination of adhesion and cohesion.

Surface tension is the elastic tendency of a fluid surface which makes it acquire the least surface area possible. It occurs at the interface between a liquid and a gas, i.e., at the liquid surface, and at the interface between two immiscible (not mixable) liquids. At liquid-air interfaces, surface tension results from the greater attraction of liquid molecules to each other (due to cohesion) than to the molecules in the air (due to adhesion). The net effect is an inward force at its surface that causes the liquid to behave as if its surface were covered with a stretched elastic membrane. Thus, the surface becomes under tension from the imbalanced forces, which is probably where the term 'surface tension' came from. Beading of rain water on a waxy surface, such as a leaf. Formation of drops occurs when a mass of liquid is stretched. Flotation of objects denser than water occurs when the object is non-wettable (insects float and stride on a water surface) and Separation of oil and water are due to the effects of surface tension.

Capillarity or capillary action, phenomenon in which the surface of a liquid is observed to be elevated or depressed where it comes into contact with a solid. For example, the surface of water in a clean drinking glass is seen to be slightly higher at the edges, where it contacts the glass, than in the middle. Capillarity can be explained by considering the effects of two opposing forces: adhesion, the attractive (or repulsive) force between the molecules of the liquid and those of the container, and cohesion, the attractive force between the molecules of the liquid (see adhesion and cohesion). Adhesion causes water to wet a glass container and thus, causes the water's surface to rise near the container's walls.

Viscosity of a fluid is a measure of its resistance to gradual deformation by shear stress or tensile stress. For liquids, it corresponds to the informal concept of 'thickness'; e.g., honey has a much higher viscosity than water. Viscosity is a property arising from collisions between neighboring particles in a fluid that are moving at different velocities. When the fluid is forced through a tube, the particles which compose the fluid generally move more quickly near the tube's axis and more slowly near its walls; therefore, some stress (such as, a pressure difference between the two ends of the tube) is needed to overcome the friction between particle layers to keep the fluid moving. For a given velocity pattern, the stress required is proportional to the fluid's viscosity. A fluid that has no resistance to shear stress is known as an ideal or inviscid fluid. Zero viscosity is observed only at very low temperatures in super fluids.

The **density** r (rho), or more strictly, mass density, of a fluid is its mass per unit volume, while the specific weight g (gamma) is its weight per unit volume. Every substance, with the one exception of water, is most dense in a solid state, second most dense in a liquid state, and least dense in a gas state. In a solid state, the molecules are packed closest together, and density is a measure of how much mass is contained in a given amount of space. Solids are so compact that their shape and volume are fixed. In a liquid state, the molecules are still close, but they have been spread apart enough to give the substance freedom to morph into any shape. So while the volume of a liquid will not increase or decrease without changes in temperature, the shape the volume makes is free to change and the molecules are free to reorganize themselves. Finally, in a gas state, the molecules are so energized and spread apart; the gas will morph into any shape and volume. Water is the only substance, i.e., denser in a liquid state than in a solid state. Liquid water is densest when it is cold (4 degrees centigrade) and salty (the greater percentage of salt the denser). As liquid water warms, it becomes less dense and as the concentration of salt is reduced is also becomes less dense. Solid water (ice) is less dense than all forms of liquid water, this is why ice floats. Finally, water in a gas state is the least dense. This is why it goes up when it evaporates and forms clouds, and why it falls down from those clouds once it becomes liquid again. Sinking and floating is a density relationship between the solid and the liquid. If the solid is less dense than the liquid, it floats. If the solid is denser than the liquid it sinks.

Elasticity is the property of solid materials to return to their original shape and size after the forces deforming them (stress) have been removed. Solid objects will deform when forces are applied on them. If the material is elastic, the object will return to its initial shape and size when these forces are removed. The physical reasons for elastic behavior can be quite different for different materials. In metals, the atomic lattice changes size and shape when forces are applied (energy is added to the system). When forces are removed, the lattice goes back to the original lower energy state. For rubbers and other polymers, elasticity is caused by the stretching of polymer chains when forces are applied. There are three types of distortions that may be produced. These are change in length, change in volume without change in shape and change of shape without change in volume. These distortions can be measured as elastic coefficient or modulus is defined as the stress divided by strain. The different modulus are Young's modulus (change in length), Bulk modulus (change in volume without change in shape) and Shear modulus (change of shape without change in volume). Solids may have all three types of distortion. Because neither liquid nor gases will support a linear strain, they have no measured values for Young's modulus. The only distortion that a fluid resists is volume change. Bulk moduli of liquids and solids are high and of the same order of magnitude. Gases are easiest to compress and hence, have the lowest Bulk modulus.

3

Electricity

DEFINITION

Electricity is defined as the production of charges.

Theories of Electricity

Fluid theory (Out dated): The theory states that electricity is weightless and invisible fluid present on all objects but capable of being distributed. If the fluid was at normal level the object was electrically neutral, but an increase in quantity of fluid gave rise to positive charge, a decrease to a negative charge. If a connection was made between two oppositely charged objects fluid passed from the positively charged object to that with a negative charge, constituting the electric current.

Electron theory (Acceptable): It states that electricity is due to flow of electron. An atom contains equal number of electrons and protons. When there is excess of electron, it is negatively charged and when there is deficiency of electron, it is positively charged. If a connection is made between a negative or positive charge, current will pass from negative to positive.

Types of Electricity

Static: It is the production of charge by rubbing the objects with each other.

The current is produced by the friction between two dissimilar materials, e.g., glass rod, silk, hair etc. (Fig. 3.1).

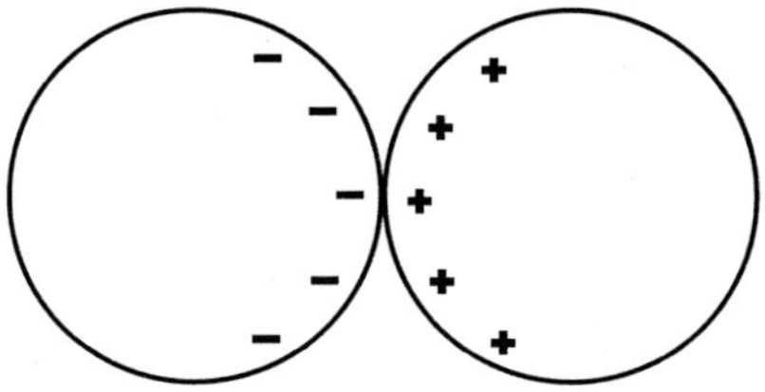

Fig. 3.1: Production of charge by rubbing the objects each other

Current: It is the flow of electron through the conducting part. Electron will flow from negative to positive whereas current will flow from positive to negative (Fig. 3.2).

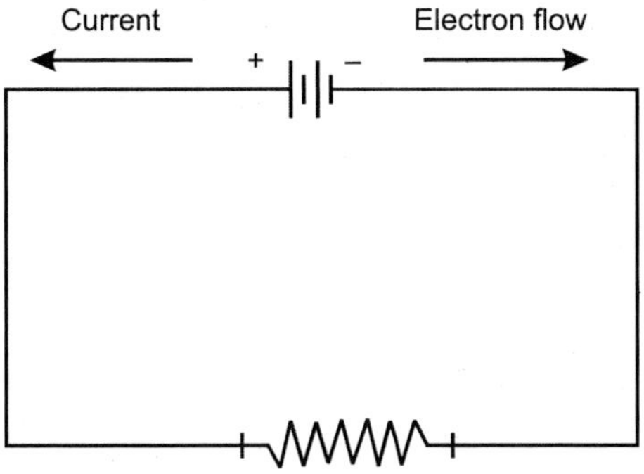

Fig. 3.2: Current flow and electron flow

PRODUCTION OF ELECTRICAL ENERGY

History

The fundamental principles of electricity generation were discovered during the 1820s and early 1830s by the British Scientist Michael Faraday. His basic method is still used today: Electricity is generated by the movement of a loop of wire, or disc of copper between the poles of a magnet.

Methods of Generating Electricity

Electricity generation is the process of generating electric power from other sources of primary energy. According to the law of conservation of energy, energy can neither be created nor be destroyed but it can be converted from one form of energy to another form.

There are seven fundamental methods of directly transforming other forms of energy into electrical energy (Table 3.1):

1. **Static electricity** from the physical separation and transport of charge (e.g., triboelectric effect and lightning). The triboelectric effect (also known as triboelectric charging) is a type of contact electrification in which certain materials become electrically charged after they come into frictional contact with a different material. For example, glass with fur, or a comb through the hair, can build up triboelectricity. The polarity and strength of the charges produced differ according to the materials, surface roughness, temperature, strain, and other properties. If a glass rod is rubbed with silk, it becomes positively charged and silk becomes negatively charged.
2. **Electromagnetic induction:** Where an electrical generator, dynamo or alternator transforms kinetic energy (energy of motion) into electricity. This is the most common used form for generating electricity and is based on Faraday's Law. Almost all commercial electrical generation is done using electromagnetic induction, in which mechanical energy forces a turbine to rotate. Turbines are commonly driven by wind, water, steam (production either by thermal power or by nuclear fission), tidal waves or burning gas like diesel. The turbine drives an electric generator.

3. **Electrochemistry:** The direct transformation of chemical energy into electricity, as in dry cell a battery used in a car, fuel cell or nerve impulse.
4. **Photovoltaic effect:** The transformation of light into electrical energy, as in solar cells.
5. **Thermoelectric effect:** The direct conversion of temperature differences to electricity, as in thermocouples, thermopiles, and thermionic converters.
6. **Piezoelectric effect:** Effect is produced from the mechanical strain of electrically anisotropic molecules or crystals.
7. **Nuclear transformation:** The creation and acceleration of charged particles (e.g., betavoltaics or alpha particle emission):

Table 3.1: Method used to generate electricity and the primary energy used

Type	*Primary energy*
Dynamo of Hydroelectric power project, Thermal power station through water, steam, wind	Kinetic energy Mechanical energy
Nuclear station	Nuclear energy
Solar energy	Radiant energy
Thermocouple	Heat or cold
Static electricity	Rubbing mechanical energy
Cells	Chemical energy

Uses of Electricity in Medicine

Therapeutic uses of electricity in medicine are called as Bioelectromagnetism. Uses can be diagnostic or therapeutic in the field of Cardiovascular, Neuromuscular and skin conditions.

Following are some of the field of applications:

- Electrotherapy
- Surgical diathermy
- Electro-acupuncture
- Cardiac pacing
- Defibrillation
- Functional electrical stimulation
- Electric implants are used for the stimulation of phrenic nerve in diaphragmatic paralysis as those seen in poliomyelitis.
- *Measurement of impedance:* Impedance plethysmography, Impedance tomography, Electrodermal response.
- ECG
- EEG
- Electrophysiological testing

Importance of Current in Physiotherapy Treatment

1. **Pain management:**
   - Relieves both acute and chronic pain thereby improving range of motion
2. **Treatment of neuromuscular dysfunction:**
   - Improvement of strength
   - Improvement of motor control
   - Retards muscle atrophy
   - Improvement of local blood flow
3. **Improves range of joint mobility:**
   - Induces repeated stretching of contracted, shortened soft tissues
4. **Tissue repair:**
   - Enhances microcirculation and protein synthesis to heal wounds
   - Increased blood flow to the injured tissues increases macrophages to clean up debris
   - Restores integrity of connective and dermal tissues
5. **Acute and chronic edema:**
   - Accelerates absorption rate
   - Affects blood vessel permeability
   - Increases mobility of proteins, blood cells and lymphatic flow
6. **Peripheral blood flow:**
   - Induces arterial, venous and lymphatic flow
7. **Iontophoresis:**
   - Delivery of pharmacological agents
   - DC (direct current) transports ions through skin
8. **Urine and fecal incontinence:**
   - Affects pelvic floor musculature to reduce pelvic pain and strengthen musculature
   - Treatment may lead to complete continence
9. **Lymphatic drainage**
   - Stimulate lymphatic system to reduce edema

Therapeutic goals and types are described in the Table 3.2.

Table 3.2: Types of electrical stimulation mode and its therapeutic goals

Type of electrical stimulation	*Goal*
Electrical muscle stimulation (EMS)	Stimulation of denervated muscle to maintain viability
Electrical stimulation for tissue repair (ESTR)	Stimulation for edema reduction, increased circulation, and wound management
Neuromuscular electrical stimulation (NMES)	Stimulation of innervated muscle to restore function including muscle strength, reduction of spasm/spasticity, prevention of atrophy, increase ROM, and muscle re-education
Functional electrical stimulation (FES)	Neural implantation for long-term muscle activation to perform functional activities
Transcutaneous electrical nerve stimulation (TENS)	Portable, superficial stimulation across the skin for pain management

4

Static Electricity

CHARGE

A charge is the fundamental property of electromagnetic force and serves as the underlying mechanism by which living cells communicate with one another. Charge is obtained by the addition or removal of electrons and is measured in coulombs (C) or microcoulombs (μC). A net gain of electrons results in negative charge, whereas a net loss of electrons results in a positive charge.

Properties of Charge

- There are two types of charge; positive and negative.
- Like charges repel while opposite attract.
- Charge is neither created nor destroyed.
- Charge can be transferred from one object to another.

Production of an Electric Charge

Charging by Friction

The simplest way of producing a static electric charge is by friction between two dissimilar materials. If a glass rod is rubbed with a piece of flannel, it will subsequently attract small pieces of paper. To demonstrate charging by friction, the materials chosen must be insulators and must be dry. Insulators do not readily allow electrons to move through them, so a charge produced on one part of the body is retained in that area. As water is a conductor of electricity and if the object is damp the charge leaks away.

Out of the following the materials nearer the head of the list gains a positive charge:

Fur, Flannel, Glass, Silk, Sealing wax

Thus, a glass rod rubbed with flannel, flannel becomes positively charged and glass rod becomes negatively charged.

Other Methods of Producing Electricity

It can be produced from dynamo, dry cell, solar cell, thermocouple, nuclear energy and piezoelectric effect. Details are already mentioned previous Chapter 3.

Characteristics of Charged Body

1. *Distribution of charge:* The charge is held on the surface of the object (superficial surface). It spreads evenly over the sphere but concentrated on the edges and corners of the flat surface (Fig. 4.1).

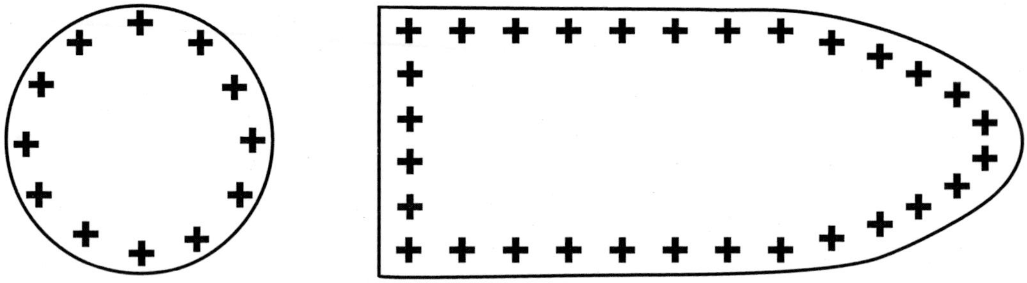

Fig. 4.1: Concentration of charge on a sphere and on a edged surface

2. *Behavior of like charges and unlike charges:* Objects with like charges repel each other whereas objects with unlike charges attract each other. For example, Silk and nylon stick each other but hair and brush move away from each other (Fig. 4.2).

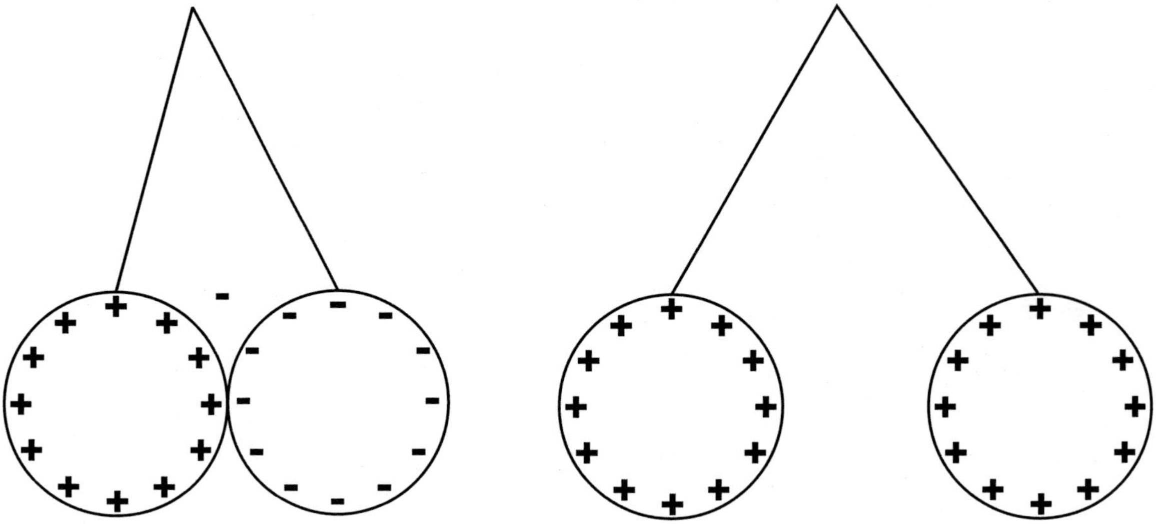

Fig. 4.2: Behavior of like charges and unlike charges

3. *Transmission of electric charge:* The charged object can produce a charge on another object by contact to produce movement of electrons (Fig. 4.3). For example, if two balls suspended on a silk thread are touched with a charged glass rod, they fly away from the rod (Fig. 4.4).

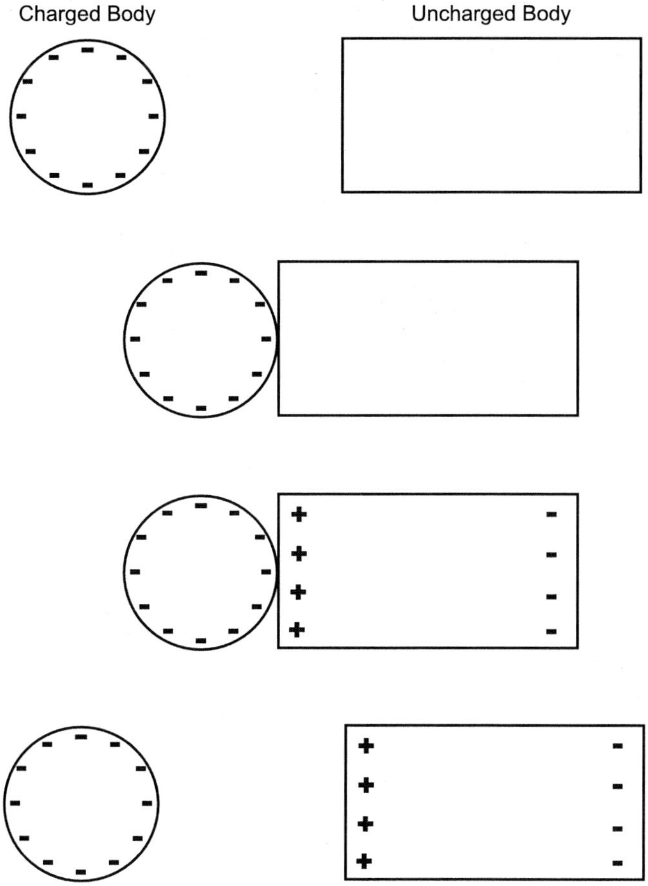

Fig. 4.3: Transmission of charge by contact

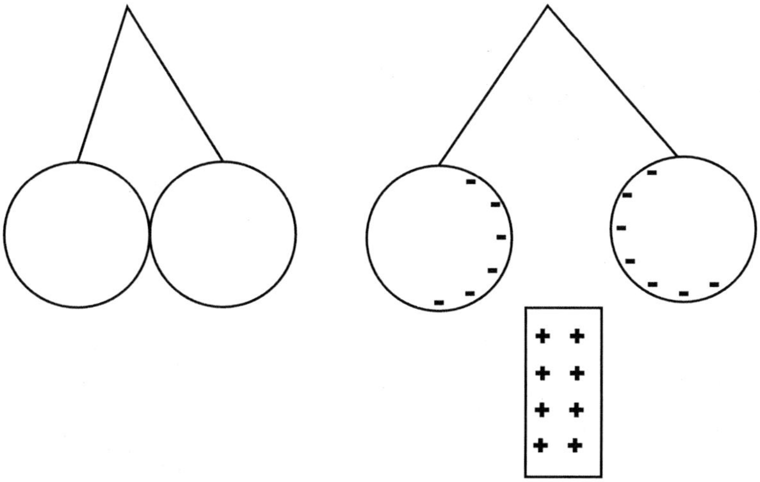

Fig. 4.4: Suspended balls fly away from charged rod

4. *Electrostatic induction:* Production of electrical or a magnetic property in one object by another without any contact between them is known as electrostatic induction (Fig. 4.5).

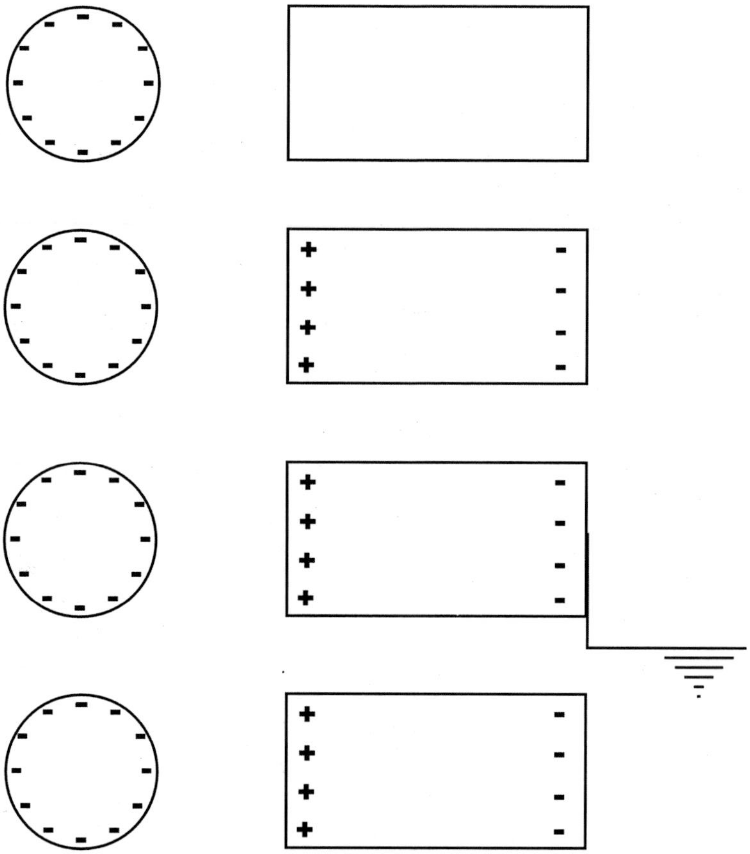

Fig. 4.5: Production of electric charge without contact

5. *Attraction of light object:* A charged object attracts an uncharged body or opposite charge, if it is sufficiently light, it moves towards the heavy object (Fig. 4.6).

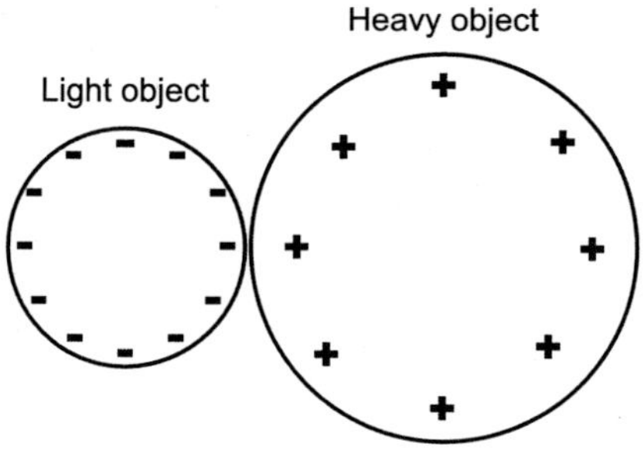

Fig. 4.6: Attraction of light object to heavy object

6. *Electric field:* Area around the charged body in which the forces resulting from the charge are present called as electric field. This is more concentrated close to the charged body (Fig. 4.7).

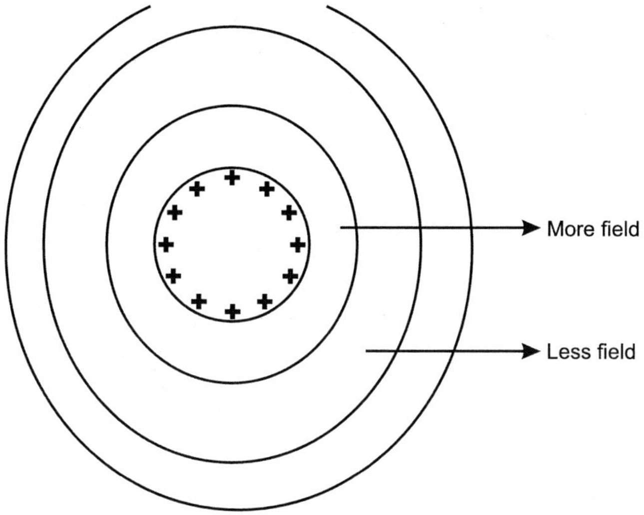

Fig. 4.7: Electric field

7. *Line of force:* The forces resulting from the charge act along definite line called as line of force (Fig. 4.8).

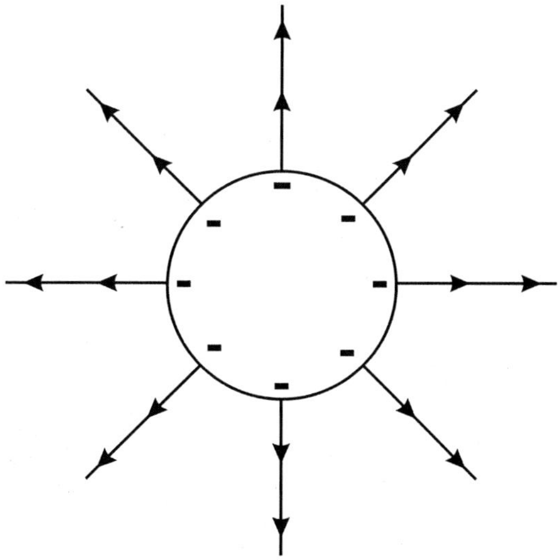

Fig. 4.8: Line of force

COULOMB'S LAW

Coulomb's law states that the magnitude of the electrostatic force of interaction between two point charges is directly proportional to the scalar multiplication of the magnitudes of charges and inversely proportional to the square of the distance between them.

The force is along the straight line joining them. If the two charges have the same sign, the electrostatic force between them is repulsive; if they have different signs, the force between them is attractive. Larger the charge or closer the two charges, the larger the attractive or repulsive forces between them.

$F \alpha (q1*q2)/r^2$

Line of Force

Definition: The force resulting from the charge act along definite line called as dynamic force.

Characteristics of Line of Force

1. It travels from negative to positive. For negative charged body, the line of force is away from it (Fig. 4.9) and for a positively charged body the line of force is towards it (Fig. 4.10).

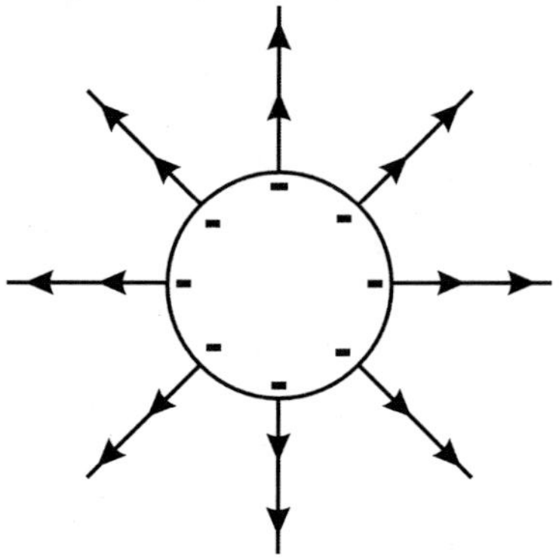

Fig. 4.9: Line of force for negatively charged body

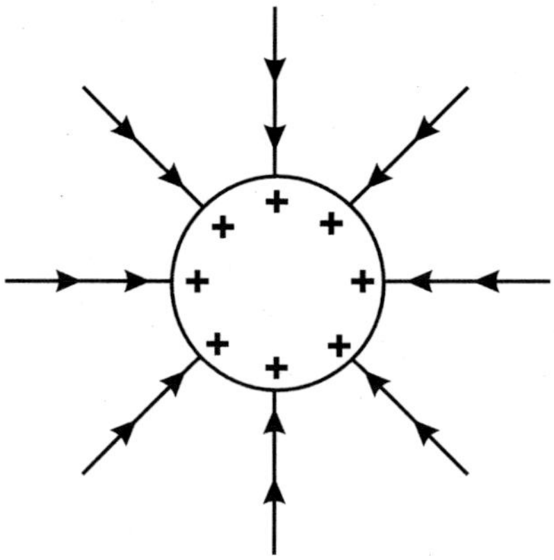

Fig. 4.10: Line of force for a positively charged body

Note: Conventionally line of force can go in opposite direction. So both ways are correct.

2. It trends to travel in straight line being a shortest distance between two points (Fig. 4.11).

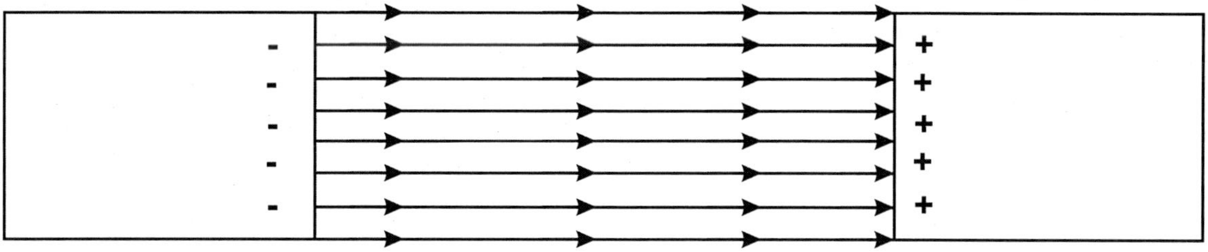

Fig. 4.11: Line of force travels in a straight line

3. Some time it may repel each other (Fig. 4.12).

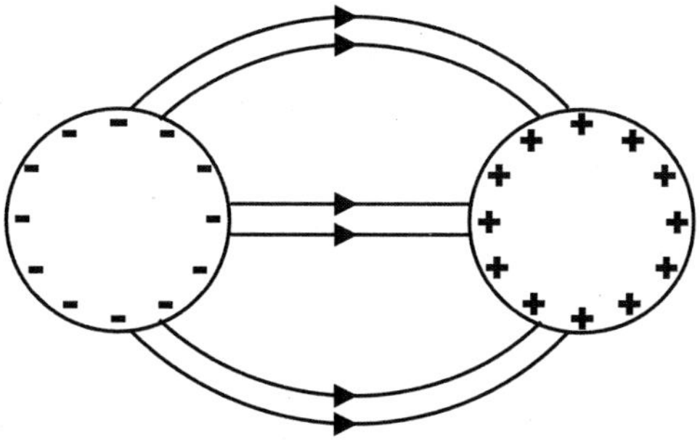

Fig. 4.12: Repelled line of force

4. It passes easily through conductors than insulators.
5. The line of force concentrates on that part of the surface of charged body nearest to the charged object over which they can exert more influence.
6. If the object is less regular line of force will concentrate on its edges (Fig. 4.13).

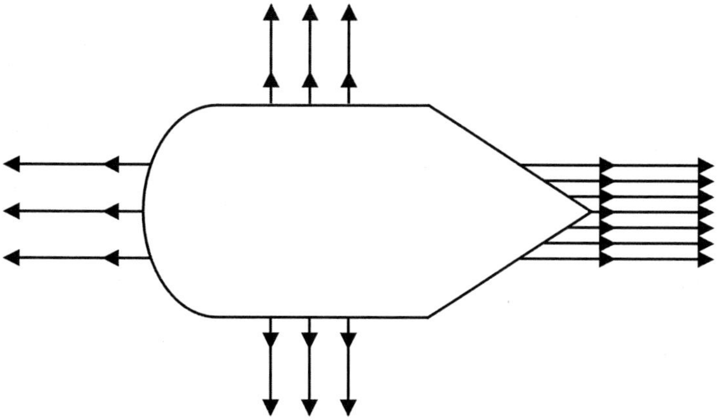

Fig. 4.13: Concentration of line of force at its edges

7. Opposite charges especially at the edges, they tend to attract each other.
8. For the same charge, the line of force tends to repel each other (Fig. 4.14).

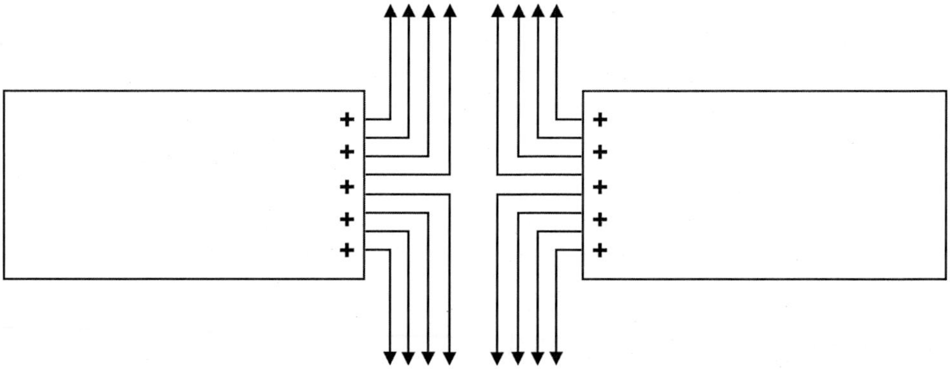

Fig. 4.14: Repulsion of line of force for same charged body

POTENTIAL AND CAPACITY

The properties exhibited by a charged body result from the stored up or potential, energy of its electric charge and its electric condition is referred to as its electrical potential. An object with excess electrons is said to be at a negative potential, one with a deficiency at a positive potential. If an object with excess electrons is connected to earth extra electrons pass from it to earth, while if one with a deficiency is connected to earth it will attract electrons from earth until it also is electrically neutral.

Factors Determining Potential

The magnitude of potential depends on:

- *The quantity of electricity with which the object is charged:* If two similar objects are charged with different quantities of electricity, the one with the most will have the greater repelling power or potential. The quantity of electricity is measured in coulombs, a coulomb being equivalent to 6.26×10^{18} electron charges.
- *The capacity of the object:* The capacity of an object is its ability to hold an electric charge and depends on the material and surface area. Charge is always on the surface so greater the surface area, greater is the capacitance of the body. Some materials hold better charge than others. So conductors have the greatest power of storing a charge.

Relationship of Electric Potential with Quantity of Charge and Capacitance

Electric potential is directly related to quantity of charge and inversely with the capacity of the object. The larger the capacitance of the body, smaller the potential or repelling power developed by a given charge. Larger the quantity of charge, larger will be the potential.

Difference of Potential

When two objects are in a different state of electric charge, a difference of potential is said to exist between them. To achieve this, one may have a negative and other a positive potential or one may with positive or negative and other may be at zero potential or both may have a charge of same nature but one be charged to a greater potential than the other. This movement of electrons constitute an electric current and is produced by force known as electromotive force. The EMF cannot produce a current unless there is a pathway or circuit through which electrons moves.

EMF and Potential Difference

EMF is total voltage in the electric circuit generated by a source or battery where as the voltage difference between any two points when the circuit is closed is called as **Potential difference**. The potential difference between two terminals of the cell is called as EMF which should be in an open circuit. Difference between EMF and potential difference is detailed in Table 4.1.

If E is the EMF of the battery used in the circuit, r is the internal resistance of circuit, R = external resistance with the intensity of current I. Then,

$E = Ir + IR$ and

$PD = E - Ir$

Table 4.1: Difference between EMF and potential difference

EMF	***Potential difference***
It transmits current both inside and outside of the cell	The potential difference current transfers between any two points in the circuit
EMF is the cause	Potential difference is result
EMF is greater than potential difference	Potential difference is less than EMF
It creates potential difference in entire circuit	Potential difference takes place between any two points in the circuit
EMF depends on internal resistance of a battery and not depends on external resistance on circuit	Potential difference depends on external resistance but does not depends on internal resistance
EMF remain constant	Does not remains constant
The part of circuit where electric energy is created from any other energy then that part contains the source of EMF	Potential difference exist in the part of the circuit where electric potential energy is transformed to any other form of energy
EMF is denoted by the symbol ε (epsilon)	It is represented by simple volt (V)
The concept of EMF is applicable only to an electric field	Potential difference is applicable to magnetic, gravitational and electric field

5

Measures of Electrical Current Flow and Its Unit

Coulomb (Q): Coulomb is the number of electrons flowing in a current. IQ = 6.25×10^8 electrons/sec.

Current (I): Current is the net movement of electrons along a conducting medium. Usually measured in milliamperes (mA: 1/1000 of an ampere) or microamperes (μA: 1/1000000 of an ampere).

Ampere (A) rate at which the electrical charge flows.

1A = 6.25×10^{18} electrons

1A = 1Q/sec

Voltage (V): Voltage is the measure of potential for current flow to occur; force resulting from an accumulation of electrons at one point in an electrical circuit. It can be high voltage or low voltage.

High voltage current: Current in which the wave form has amplitude of greater than 150 V with relatively short-pulse duration.

Low voltage current: Current in which the waveform has amplitude of less than 150 V.

Volt: The unit of PD and is the amount of work required to move a coulomb of charge.

Wattage

Relationship between voltage and ampere (P) used to designate the power of current.

Power (W): Power is defined as the amount of work being performed in a unit of time.

1 Watt: The power produced by 1 ampere of current flowing with the force of 1V

P = 120 V × 2 A

= 240 Watt

Ohm (Ω): Ohm is the unit of measure that indicates resistance to current flow; materials resistance to the movement of electrons.

1 ohm: The amount of resistance needed to develop 0.24 calories of heat when 1A of current is applied for 1 sec.

RESISTANCE AND IMPEDANCE

Resistance is a concept used for DC (direct currents) whereas impedance is the AC (alternating current) equivalent.

Resistance (R): Opposition to electrons flow in a conducting material when DC is applied.

Impedance (Z): The effective resistance of an electric circuit or component to alternating current, arising from the combined effects of ohmic resistance and reactance.

Reactance (Y): It is the inverse of Impedance. So Reactance Y = 1/Z. It tells us the quickness with which any change in input voltage the circuit will react. So lower Impedance means, larger will be Reactance. Reactance can arise from the effect of inductance or capacitance or both and causing the current to be out of phase with the electromotive force causing it.

Inductance (I): Degree that a varying current can induce voltage (H – Henry) (negligible in biological spectrum).

Capacitance (C): Frequency dependent ability to store a charge (C), many of the cell membranes is capacitors.

Table 5.1: Summary of units of electrical current flow

AMPERE
It is that unvarying strength current which when flowing through two straight parallel wire placed 1m apart in a vacuum produces between them a force of 2×10^{-7} Newton per meter of their length
FARADAY
It is the capacity of an object which is charged to a potential of 1 volt by 1 coulomb of electricity. In practice, this is a very large unit so the microfarad (μF) is commonly used
$1\ \mu F = 10^{-6} F$
VOLT
That EMF which when applied to a conductor with a resistance of 1 ohm produces a current of 1A
COULOMB
It is the quantity of electricity which passes any given point in a circuit when a current of 1A flows for 1 sec, it is equivalent to 6.26×10^{18}4 electrons
WATT
A unit of power being a rate of work of 1 J/sec.

6

Flow of Electricity in Solid, Liquid and Gases

INTRODUCTION

A transmission medium is a material substance (solid, liquid, gas, or plasma) that can propagate energy waves. For example, the transmission medium for sounds is usually air, but solids and liquids may also act as transmission media for sound. The absence of a material medium in vacuum may also constitute a transmission medium for electromagnetic waves, such as, light and radio waves. While material substance is not required for electromagnetic waves to propagate, such waves are usually affected by the transmission media they pass through, for instance, by absorption or by reflection or refraction at the interfaces between media.

In Solids

On the basis of electric behavior, the solids can be classified into three categories. They are conductors, insulators and semiconductors.

In solid conductors like metals, the valence electrons of the atoms do not remain attached to individual atoms but are free to move throughout the volume of the conductor without altering its physical properties. Under the effect of an external electric field, the valence electrons move in a definite direction causing electric current in the conductors. Thus, the electrons are the carriers of electricity in solid conductors.

In insulators, it takes a great deal of energy to cause electrons to move from one atom to another and if they do so, it alters the structure or nature of the material. The distinction between conductors and insulators is such that some electrons in conductors are able to accept the small amounts of energy available from an electric field to alter their energy level and move out of position whereas electrons in insulators need vastly more energy to reach the necessary energy level for movement within the material.

Semiconductors are the materials which exhibit the characteristics of an insulator but have some electrons which can behave as electrons in a conductor. Intrinsic semiconductors have a small number of free electrons at room temperature. Extrinsic semiconductors achieve the same characteristics by the addition of very small quantities of some other element. Adding a very small amount of phosphorous to silicon converts into extrinsic semiconductor is called as doping.

In Liquids

On the basis of electric behavior, the liquids can be classified into three categories. They are insulators, conductors and electrolytes.

Liquids like vegetable oil, distilled water do not allow the current to pass through them. Mercury is a liquid metal which allows the current to pass through them but do not dissociate into ions. Some solutions like salts, acid and bases dissociate into ions while allowing the current to pass through them.

In Gases

Normally, the gases are insulators of electricity. But, they can be ionized by applying a high potential difference at low pressures or by their exposures to X-rays. The ionized gas contains positive ions and electrons. Thus, positive ions and electrons are the carriers of electricity.

In Vacuum

In vacuum, there is no retarding force on any charged particle with constant velocity. To this extent, no extra work is required in maintaining a constant current through any surface in vacuum. The resistance of the vacuum is in fact, infinite. So, they may act as insulators since they do not have charge carriers. To flow electron across a vacuum, you need a force to get the electrons to travel across the vacuum. Cathode Ray tube is an example for flow of electrons through vacuum. In a CRT, the cathode is heated, which gives the electrons the energy they need to escape the cathode. A large electric field then accelerates the free electrons across the vacuum and onto a target (screen). In this case, other fields are also used to steer the beam to get an optimal picture. If you have a different system – imagine an anode and a cathode in a vacuum separated by a small distance – with no deliberate heating taking place – then the potential difference (i.e., potential energy or voltage) between the two electrodes must be large enough that the electrons can 'leap' between them. They need to leap because the vacuum is a perfect insulator and so there is no medium in which they can flow (like through a metal conductor) so they must acquire all of the energy necessary to cover the distance before they can escape the cathode. Larger gap to be traversed implies larger potential difference required to get the electrons to make the leap.

7

Effects of Electric Current

Effects of electrical current include thermal, electric and magnetic effects.

THERMAL EFFECT

When a current is passed through a conductor, a part of electrical energy is converted into heat and it is liberated according to Joule's law.

Joule's law states that the amount of heat produced in a conductor is proportional to square of the intensity of current, the resistance and the time for which the current flows. As electrical energy is converted into heat, work is done and the amount of heat produced depends on the amount of work done.

Work done = watts × time

= E × I × t joules

Where,

E = EMF measured in volts

I = Intensity of current measured in amperes

T = Time measured in seconds

By Ohm's law,

E = I × R

So, work done = I × R × I × t

$$\textbf{Work done} = \mathbf{I^2\,Rt}$$

One calorie of heat is produced by 4.2 joules of work

So, heat generated = I^2 Rt/4.2

Application of Joule's Law in Physiotherapy

As resistance is wired in series with each other, the intensity and time is same for all parts of the circuit. As the heat generated is directly proportional to the resistance, more heat is produced in high resistance than a lower one. When resistances are wired in parallel with each other, time is same for all parts of the circuit but the intensity is inversely proportional to resistance. As the lower resistance has higher intensity, more heat is generated in a lower resistance compared to higher resistance. In series connection, heat generated is dependent on resistance whereas in parallel heat generated depends on the intensity. In case of UVR or IRR, the lamp is in series with supply wires. The resistance of supplying the wire is small compared to that of the filament of the lamp. Therefore, there is more heating effect in the filament of lamp than that in the supply wires (practically it is unheated). A fuse wire is made up of tin and lead has high resistance and low melting point. It is in series with electrical installations and protects them from the strong currents.

CHEMICAL EFFECTS

Chemical effects are produced when a direct current is passed through an electrolyte; the procedure is known as electrolysis. An electrolyte is a substance which contains ions. The molecules of the electrovalent compounds consist entirely of ions, hence, they are strong electrolytes. Covalent compounds have weak dissociation of molecules, hence they are weak electrolytes. The properties of electrolyte become more apparent when the substance is dissolved in water as there is more room for ions to move than when it is in solid form. Sodium chloride, is a strong electrolyte, so when it is dissolved in water the solution contains positive sodium ions, negative chlorine ions, positive hydrogen ions, negative hydroxyl ions and water molecules. When ions are neutralized at the electrodes chemical changes takes place. For a solution like sodium chloride, positive sodium and hydrogen ions migrate to cathode and negative chlorine and hydroxyl ions migrate to anode. In cathode, hydrogen is lower than sodium in the electrochemical series, so its ions are more easily neutralized. The hydrogen is given up as bubbles and hydroxyl ion concentration rises and reaction is alkaline. In anode chlorine ions are neutralized, and then it reacts with water to form hydrochloric and hypochlorous acids. So, the reaction is acidic.

Faraday's Law of Electrolysis

First Law: According to this law, *the chemical deposition due to flow of current through an electrolyte is directly proportional to the quantity of electricity (coulomb) passed through it, i.e., mass of chemical deposition,*

$$m \propto \text{Quantity of electricity, } Q \Rightarrow m = Z.Q$$

Where Z is a constant of proportionality and is known as electrochemical equivalent of the substance. If we put Q = 1 coulomb in the above equation, we will get Z = m which implies that electrochemical equivalent of any substance is the amount of the substance deposited on passing of 1 coulomb through its solution. This constant of passing of electrochemical equivalent is generally expressed in terms of milligram per coulomb or kilogram per coulomb.

Second Law: It states that, *when the same quantity of electricity is passed through several electrolytes, the mass of the substances deposited are proportional to their respective chemical equivalent or equivalent weight.*

The chemical equivalent or equivalent weight of a substance can be determined by Faraday's laws of electrolysis and it is defined as the weight of that substance which will combine with or displace unit weight of hydrogen. The chemical equivalent of hydrogen is, thus, unity. Since valency of a substance is equal to the number of hydrogen atoms, the chemical equivalent of a substance, therefore, may be defined as the ratio of its atomic weight to its valency. Valency of an element is a measure of its combining power with other atoms when it forms chemical compounds or molecules.

Thus,

$$Chemical\ equivalent = \frac{Atomic\ Weight}{Valency}$$

If z is electrochemical equivalent and E is the chemical equivalent according to Faraday's second law, z is directly proportional to E

E = Fz, where, F is the Faraday's constant, F = E/z

F = E/m/q

= qE/m

MAGNETIC EFFECT OF AN ELECTRIC CURRENT

An electric current sets up a magnetic field around the conductor through which it is passing. This can be demonstrated by holding a wire carrying a current over and parallel to a compass needle, for as the current flows the needle is deflected to one side, indicating the presence of magnetic forces. The direction of deflection of magnetic needle is reversed if the deflection of current in the wire is reversed. The direction of deflection of magnetic needle can be easily determined by **SNOW rule**. According to **SNOW rule**, when current flows through a conductor from South to North direction and the wire is held over magnetic needle then the north pole of the magnetic needle deflects towards west and vice versa (Fig. 7.1).

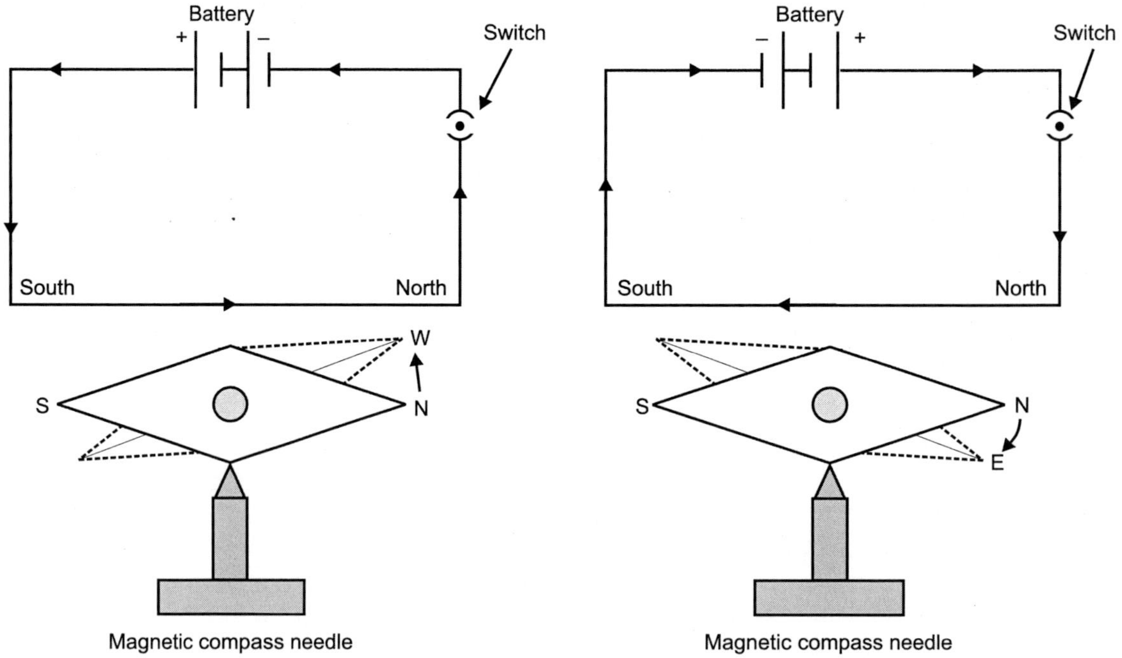

Fig. 7.1: SNOW rule; deflection of compass needle

The magnetic field around the conductor consists of a number of concentric closed lines of force (Fig. 7.2).

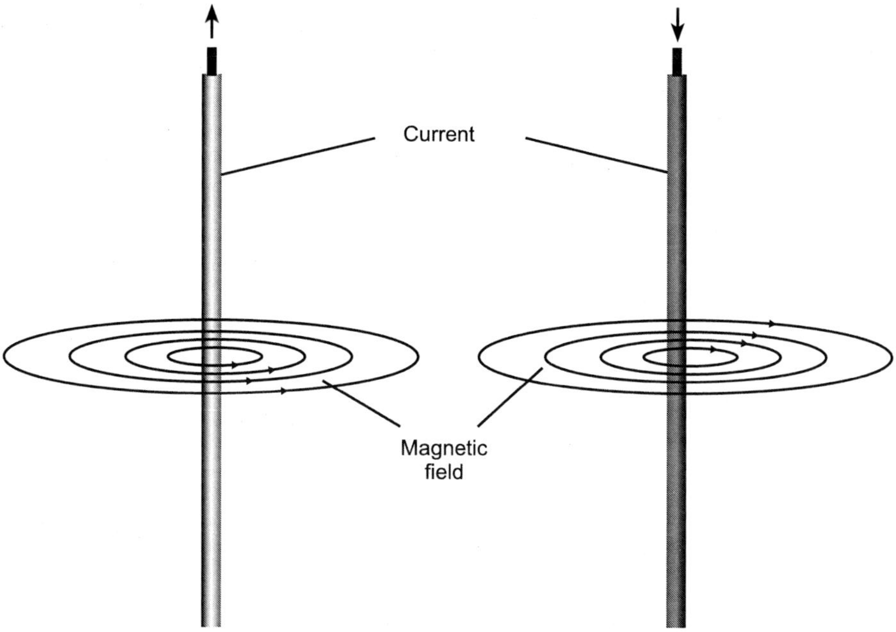

Fig. 7.2: Direction of current flow and the magnetic field

From the Figure 7.2, it is noted that when current flows through the conductor in upward direction, the direction of circular magnetic lines are anti-clockwise if we observe from the top. On the other hand, if the current flows through the conductor in downward direction, the circular magnetic lines are clockwise if we observe from the top.

Properties of magnetic field due to a current carrying conductor can be summarized as below:

All lines of magnetic field are circular in shape, symmetrical to each other and concentric with the axis of current carrying conductor.

The radius of the lines of force increases as we go away from the axis of the conductor.

The direction of magnetic circular line depends upon the direction of flow of current through the conductor.

The magnetic flux density of the induced magnetic field around the conductor increases if the current flowing through the conductor is increased and it decreases if the current is decreased.

The direction of this magnetic field of current carrying conductor can be determined by Cork Screw rule or Right Hand rule.

Maxwell's Cork Screw Rule

If the right-handed cork screw is held with its axis parallel to the conductor pointing the direction of flow of current and the head of the screw is rotated in such a direction that the screw moves in the direction of flow of current, then the direction in which the head of screw is rotated, will be the direction of magnetic lines of force.

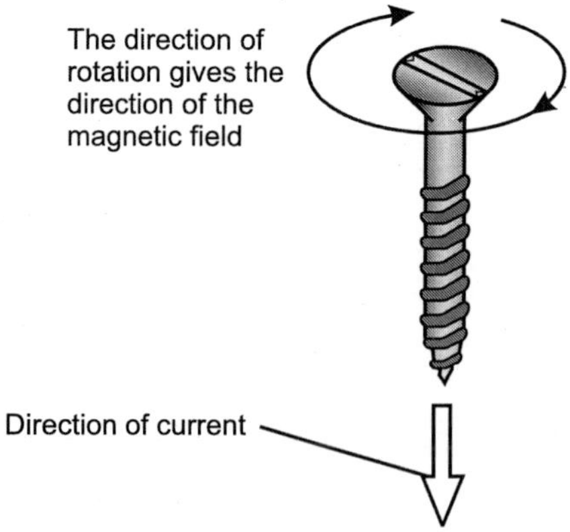

Fig. 7.3: Maxwell's cork screw rule

Right Hand Thumb Rule

If the current carrying conductor is held in right hand by the observer so that it is encircled by fingers stretching the thumb at right to the fingers in the direction of flow of current then finger tips will point the direction of magnetic lines of force (Fig. 7.4).

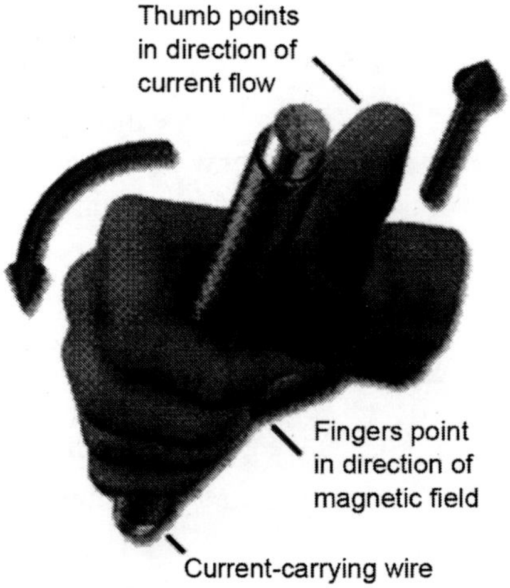

Fig. 7.4: Right hand rule

Magnetic Flux Density Due to a Current Carrying Conductor

The Biot-Savart Law relates magnetic fields to the currents which are their sources. In a similar manner, Coulomb's law relates electric fields to the point charges which are their sources.

As per Biot-Savart law, the expression of **magnetic flux density** at a point P nearer to a conductor carrying a current 'I' is given as,

$$dB = dB = \frac{\mu}{4\pi} \frac{I \,.\, dL \,.\, \sin\theta}{r^2}$$

Where, dB is the infinitesimal flux density at point P.

Current I is passing through the conductor.

dl is infinitesimal length of conductor.

r is the radius vector from center of element dl to point P.

θ is the angle between current and radius vector.

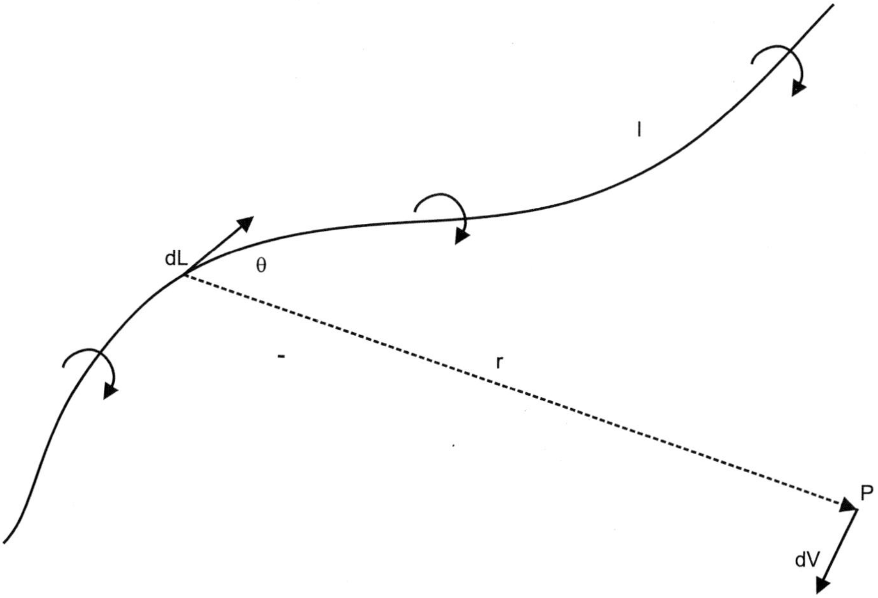

Fig. 7.5: Description of Biot-Savarts law

Factors which influence force exerted by a moving charge in a magnetic field:

- The magnitude of the force F experienced is directly proportional to the magnitude of the charge.
- The magnitude of the force F is directly proportional to the component of velocity acting perpendicular to the direction of magnetic field.
- The magnitude of the force F is directly proportional to the magnitude of the magnetic field applied.

8

Magnet

DEFINITION

Magnet is the substance which shows certain properties like power of attraction for certain materials and tendency, when free to rotate to come to rest pointing in a north-south direction.

Molecular Theory of Magnetism

No matter how many times a magnet is divided, it always presents a north and south pole. This property is carried at molecular level. In non-magnetize stage, the molecular magnets are disordered (Fig. 8.1a). In magnetize stage, it is ordered (Fig. 8.1b). In permanent magnet, the friction between molecules is more so ordering is more retained. In temporary magnet, the friction is less so the molecules are disordered. Heating or hammering will lose the properties. The common substances which show magnetic properties are iron, nickel, cobalt. They all lie next to each other in the periodic table.

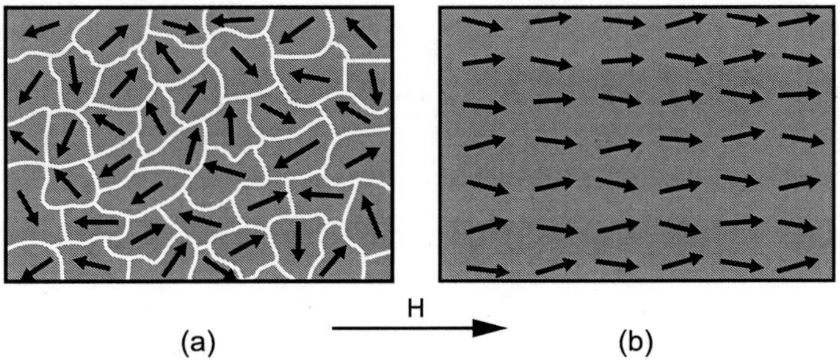

Fig. 8.1: Ordered and disordered stages

Classification of Magnet

- *Natural Magnet:* (Iodestone)

  It is type of iron ore with magnetic property.

- *Artificial magnet:* Produce magnetic properties in certain materials like iron, steel, nickel and cobalt.
- *Temporary magnet:* The material which readily acquired magnetic property and loss this property very quickly is called temporary magnet, e.g., soft iron.
- *Permanent magnet:* It is difficult to magnetize but retains this property for longer period, e.g., steel.
- *Electromagnet:* If the current pass through coil of wire, it produces magnetic properties.

Based on the shape, it is divided into bar magnet, ring magnet and horse shoe magnet (Fig. 8.2).

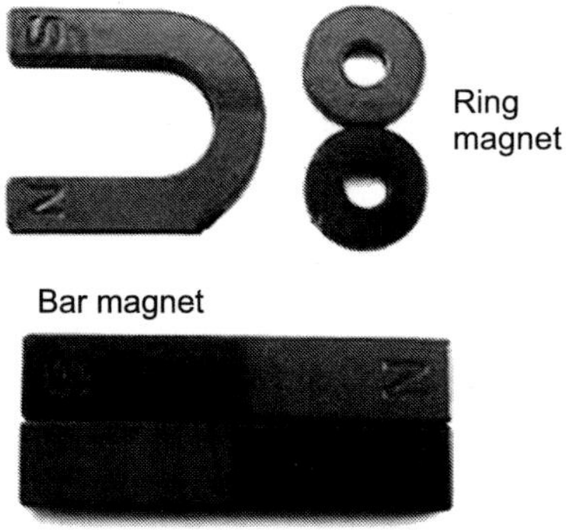

Fig. 8.2: Types of magnet

Properties of Magnet

Sitting in a north-south direction: When a magnet is free to rotate, it comes to rest with one end pointing towards the magnetic north pole of the earth (north pole), the other point towards south pole of the earth.

Behavior of like and unlike poles: Like poles repel each other and unlike poles attract each other (Fig. 8.3).

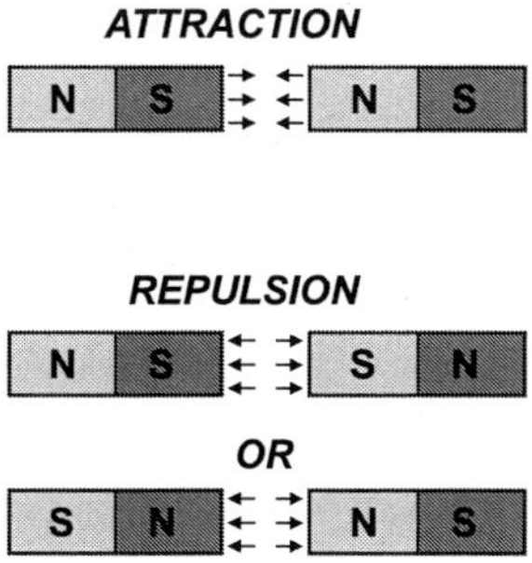

Fig. 8.3: Behavior of like and unlike poles

Transmission of properties by contact or induction:

Magnetization by contact: Stroke a piece of iron with one pole of a bar magnet. Stroke should be carried in same direction. The end of the piece of the material at which the stroke commences, assumes the same polarity as of the pole which is stroked. When the stroke finishes pole assumes the opposite polarity. That is in the iron piece starting side will assume same pole as that of the magnet and ending side opposite pole is achieved (Fig. 8.4).

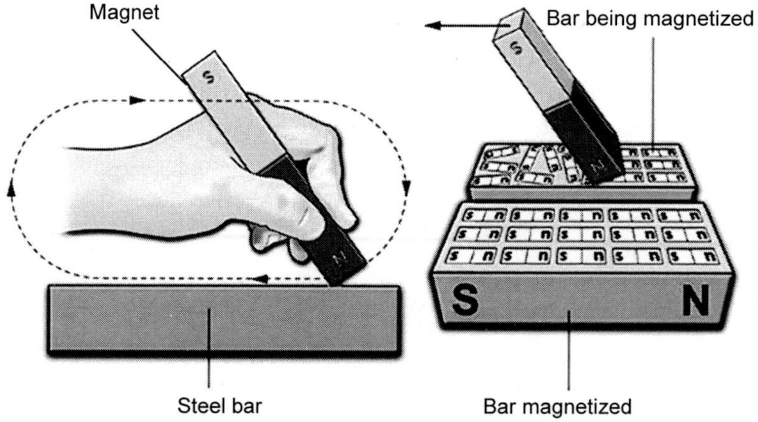

Fig. 8.4: Magnetisation by contact

Magnetization by induction: Magnetic induction is defined as production of magnetic properties in one object by another without contact in between them (Fig. 8.5).

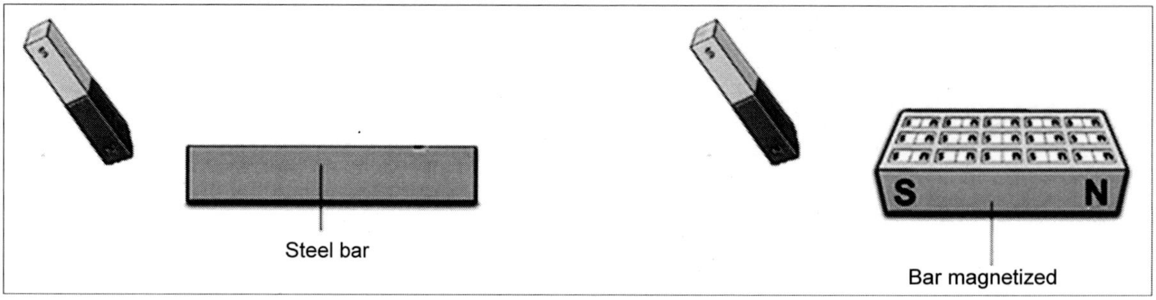

Fig. 8.5: Magnetization by induction

Attraction for objects of magnetizable material:

Magnet has the property of attracting object of a magnetizable material. Hence, there is always tendency of light objects materials to get attracted towards the magnet.

MAGNETIC FIELD

Area around a magnet in which magnetic forces are apparent is called as magnetic field. The magnetic forces act along definite line and these are the lines along which a free north pole will travel if they will be able to move the magnetic field.

Properties of Magnetic Line of Force (Figs. 8.6 and 8.7)

1. **It travels away from North and towards South pole**
2. **It tends to take shortest pathway between two coils**

3. **The magnetic line of force tends to repel each other**
4. **It travels more easy through magnetizable materials**

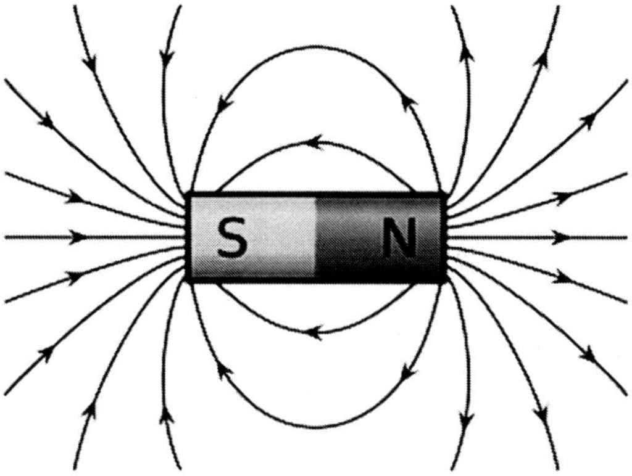

Fig. 8.6: Magnetic field around single magnet

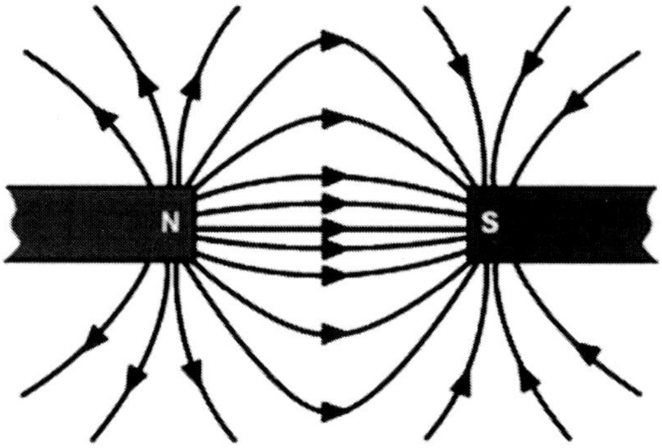

Fig. 8.7: Magnetic field between two magnets

9

Conductors and Insulators

DIFFERENTIATION

Electrons can move in a current only if there is a relatively easy pathway to move along. Materials that permit this free movement of electrons are referred to as **conductors**. **Conductance** is a term that defines the ease with which current flows along a conducting medium and is measured in units called siemens. Metals (copper, gold, silver, aluminum) are good conductors of electricity, as are electrolyte solutions, because both are composed of large numbers of free electrons that are given up readily. Thus, materials that offer little opposition to current flow are good conductors.

Materials that resist current flow are called **insulators**. Insulators contain relatively fewer free electrons, and thus, offer greater resistance to electron flow. Air, wood, and glass are all considered insulators. The number of amperes flowing in a given conductor is dependent both on the voltage applied and on the conduction characteristics of the material.

Resistance: The conductor through which electrons have to flow offers some resistance to their flow.

Factors which influences the resistance:

- *The material of the conductor:* A good conductor has least resistance where as poor conductor has high resistance.
- *The length of the pathway:* Longer the pathway, greater is the electrical resistance.
- *The cross-sectional area of the conductor:* The greater the cross-sectional area, resistance will be lower.
- *Temperature:* As temperature of the conductor increases more the kinetic movement of the molecules. This increased movement impedes the passage of the electrons and so increases the resistance.

Magnitude of Current

The intensity or magnitude of current (I) is the rate of flow of electrons through the conductor per second. The magnitude of a current depends upon the applied EMF and resistance of the conductor. The greater the EMF applied, the greater is the flow of electrons, hence, there is direct relationship. The greater the resistance, more difficult it is for the electrons to move through the conductor, so a high resistance tends to produce a low current, hence, there is a inverse relationship.

10

Resistance in Series and Parallel, Its Application to Physiotherapy

RESISTANCE IN SERIES

In the Figure 10.1, the individual resistance R_1, R_2, R_3 are connected in series in a circuit with a voltage V. The resistance are connected together end to end so that current has only one point. The current has to compulsory pass through each of the resistance. Total resistance is equal to sum of individual resistance. Intensity of current is same throughout the circuit. Potential drop across each resistance is directly proportional to the resistance.

Then

$$V/I = R$$

$$R = R_1 + R_2 + R_3$$

$$V = I\,(R_1 + R_2 + R_3)$$

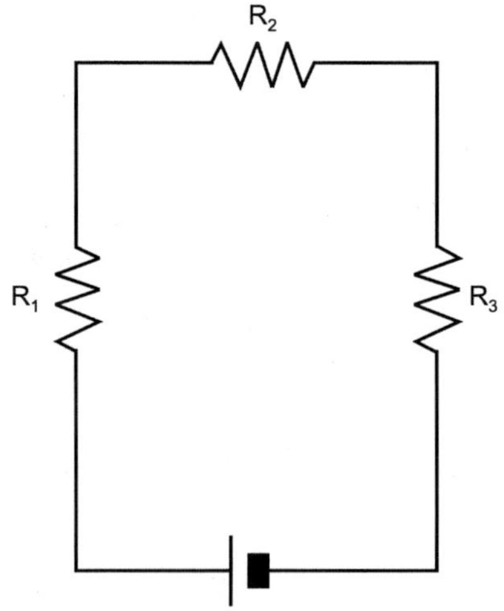

Fig. 10.1: Resistance in series

Resistance in Parallel

In the Figure 10.2, the individual resistance: R_1, R_2, R_3 are connected in parallel in a circuit with a voltage V. The resistance are connected so that they tap the main circuit at two points. This provides the alternating pathway for the current. As the pathway is taken from same two points on the circuit, potential drop across all of them is equal. The intensity of the current in each of pathway is inversely proportional to the each resistance of pathway. Total resistance is less than that of its individual resistance.

Then,

$I = V/R$

$I = V/R_1 + V/R_2 + V/R_3$

$I/R = I/R_1 + I/R_2 + I/R_3$

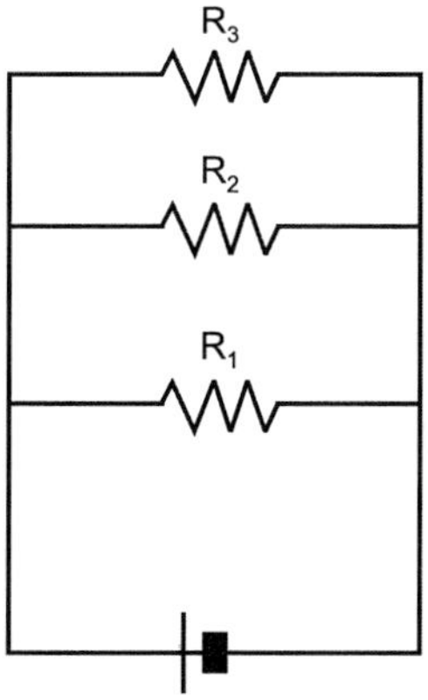

Fig. 10.2: Resistance in parallel

APPLICATION OF SERIES AND PARALLEL RESISTANCE IN ELECTRO-THERAPY

1. Voltmeter is always connected in parallel and Ammeter is always connected in series in a circuit (Fig. 10.3).

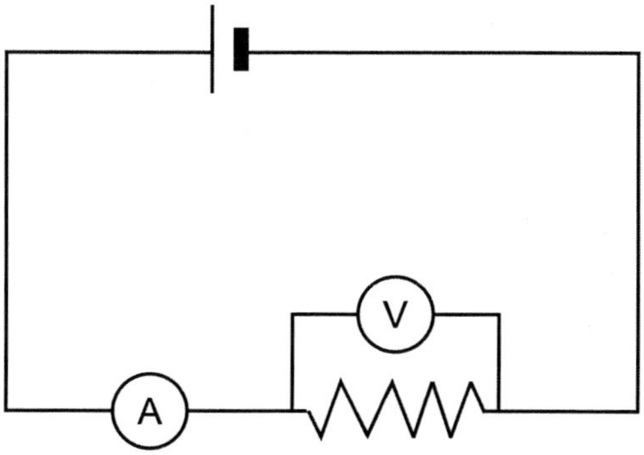

Fig. 10.3: Connection of ammeter and voltmeter to a circuit

2. *Current flow in tissue:* With electrical stimulation, the current passes to the tissue through skin and fat from the electrode. This passage through the skin is a series circuit. The total resistance to the current flow is the sum of the resistances at the site of electrode, i.e., skin and fat. After the current passes through the skin and fat, it comes in contact with a number of different types of tissues like bone, connective tissue, blood, muscle. This is a parallel circuit. The current has different pathways to choose to reach finally to the muscle. The total current travelling through these tissues is the sum of the currents in each different type of the tissue. So, the total resistance will be less as current may travel through the least resistance.

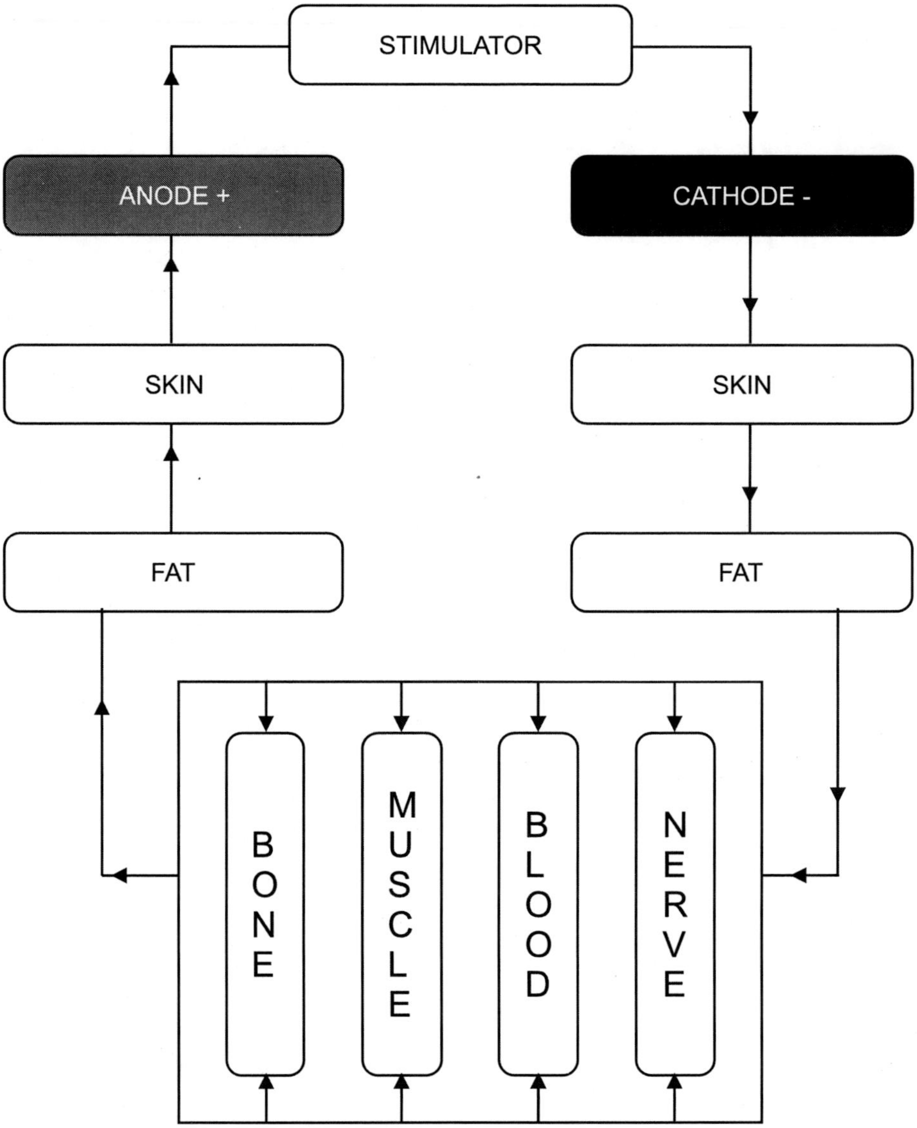

Fig. 10.4: Current flow in the tissue

3. Devices for regulating the intensity of current.
   - *Series rheostat or variable resistance:* The wire from the one end of the resistance coil connected to the source of supply, the other end is connected to patient circuit. Thus, the coil is in series with circuit (Fig. 10.5).

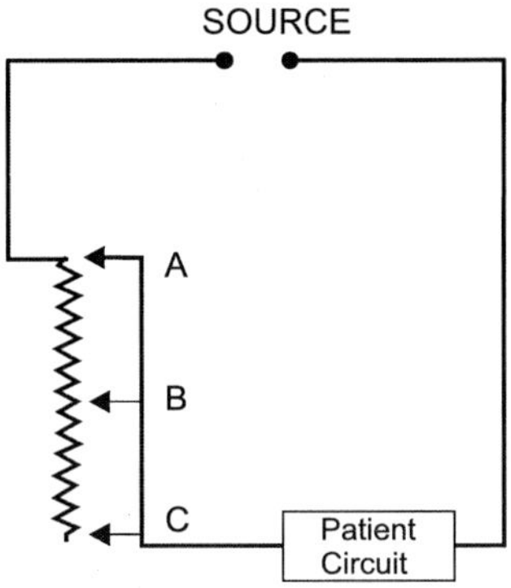

Fig. 10.5: Series rheostat

When the contact is in lower side of coil, full resistance included and the current is minimal (Point C). When the contact reaches the upper hand side, the resistance is minimum and intensity is maximum (Point A). If it is mid point (Point B) moderate intensity is achieved.

This setup is suitable for UV lamps, Infrared lamps, Laser, etc. It is not used in stimulator because the intensity never reduces to zero so as soon as the apparatus is turned on patient receives a shock.

- *Potentiometer (potential divider/shunt rheostat):* The two ends of the coil are connected to source of supply. The circuit in which the current is to be regulated is taken parallel to the coil by one wire from one end of coil; the other wire is at sliding contact (Fig. 10.6).
  - In point A the two wires of parallel circuit are in contact so intensity is zero
  - In point C the least resistance and more current
  - In point B more resistance and least current
  - This setup is used for stimulator where intensity is reduced to zero. So, it is used in electrical stimulation, TENS and IFT.

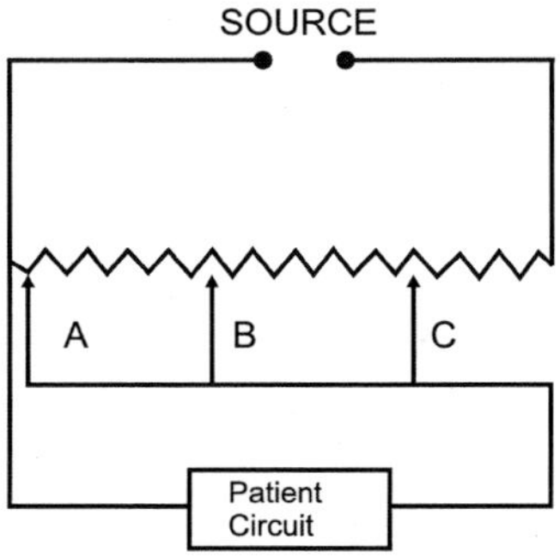

Fig. 10.6: Shunt rheostat

11

Ohm's Law and Its Application to DC and AC Currents, Application to Physiotherapy

OHM'S LAW

It states that, *the current in an electric circuit is directly proportional to voltage and inversely proportional to resistance.*

$I \alpha V/R$,

Where, I is the current, V is the voltage, R is the resistance

An analogy comparing the movement of water with the movement of electricity may help to clarify this relationship among current flow, voltage, and resistance (Table 11.1). In order for water to flow, some type of pump must create a force to produce movement. Likewise, the volt is the pump that produces the electron flow. The resistance to water flow is dependent on the length, diameter, and smoothness of the water pipe. The resistance to electrical flow depends on the characteristics of the conductor. The amount of water flowing is measured in gallons, whereas the amount of electricity flowing is measured in amperes.

Table 11.1: Electron flow *versus* water flow

Electron Flow is Analogous to Water Flow	
Electron flow	Water flow
Volt	Pump
Ampere	Gallon
Ohm (Property of conductor)	Resistance (Length and distance of pipe)

Application of Ohm's Law to AC and DC

Ohm's law to AC is different from Ohm's law to DC. Because DC circuit has only pure resistance whereas AC circuit may contain inductor (coil), capacitance (capacitor) and resistance (resistor). This circuit will affect the phase of the voltage and current. So, the phase shift must be taken into account when analysing the circuit.

Analysing resistance in DC

For a 50 volts in circuit with 5 Ohm's resistance, the net current is as follows:

$I = V/R = 50/5 = 10$ A

Analysing resistance in AC

In an AC circuit with 50 volts, the resistor with 5 ohms, inductor with 25 Henry and capacitance is 15 farad.

The net impedance (X) = inductance – capacitance

$$X = X_L - X_C$$
$$= 25 - 15$$
$$= 10$$

The net resistance (R) $= \sqrt{r^2 + X^2}$

$$= \sqrt{5^2 + 10^2}$$
$$= \sqrt{125}$$
$$= 11.2$$

So, the net current is

$$I = V/R$$
$$= 50/11.2$$
$$= 4.46 \text{ A}$$

From the above calculation, it is understood that with 50 volts and resistance of 5 ohms, the net current flow in a DC circuit is 10 A and in an AC circuit it is 4.46 A.

Limitations of Ohm's Law

1. This law cannot be applied to unilateral networks. A unilateral network has unilateral elements like diode, transistors, etc., which do not have same voltage current relation for both directions of current.
2. Ohm's law is also not applicable for non-linear elements. Non-linear elements are those which do not give current through it, is not exactly proportional to the voltage applied, that means the resistance value of those elements changes for different values of voltage and current. Examples of non-linear elements are thyristor, electric arc, etc.
3. Temperature: As resistance varies with temperature.
4. It is not applicable for a gaseous conductor.
5. It is not applicable to semiconductors like germanium and silicon.
6. It cannot apply to a conducting body when its shape is deformed.

Application of Ohm's Law in Physiotherapy

- It helps us in determining; voltage, current or resistance of a linear circuit when the other two quantities are known to us.
- It makes power calculation a lot simpler, like when we know the value of the resistance for a particular circuit, we need not know both the current and the voltage to calculate the power dissipation since P = VI. Rather we can use Ohm's law.

  According to Ohm's law $I = V/R$, so, $P = V^2/R$
- Constant current versus Constant voltage stimulator (described below).

Constant Current Stimulators produce a constant current independent of resistance encountered. The voltage adjusts to maintain constant current flow. The advantage of this type of stimulator is to ensure a consistency physiologic response during the treatment. The negative is potential pain when the voltage increases to overcome resistance.

Constant Voltage Stimulators, conversely, produce a constant voltage. The current adjusts to depending on changes in resistance. This unit is advantageous in preventing discomfort with changes in resistance, such as, an electrode losing full contact, but quality of response can be decreased with these automatic resistance changes.

To determine constant current versus constant voltage on an electrical stimulation unit, slowly start to peel one electrode off the skin while the machine is on. If the current sharpens, the machine is constant current; if the current lessens, the machine is constant voltage when the electrode is being peeled away.

12

Condenser or Capacitor

DEFINITION

It is a device used to store electric charge.

Principle

Based on the principle of static electricity. If the charged conductor is brought to another conductor its store increases especially if the other conductor holds the opposite electric charge.

Basic Properties of Condenser

- It accumulates electric charge.
- It blocks DC and passes AC.
- Higher the frequency or higher the capacitance, more easily the current can pass.

Construction

A capacitor consists of metal sheets and space between them is occupied by dielectric medium which is a layer of insulating material. A capacitor with large capacity consists of a series of metal sheets which are separated by dielectric media (Fig. 12.1).

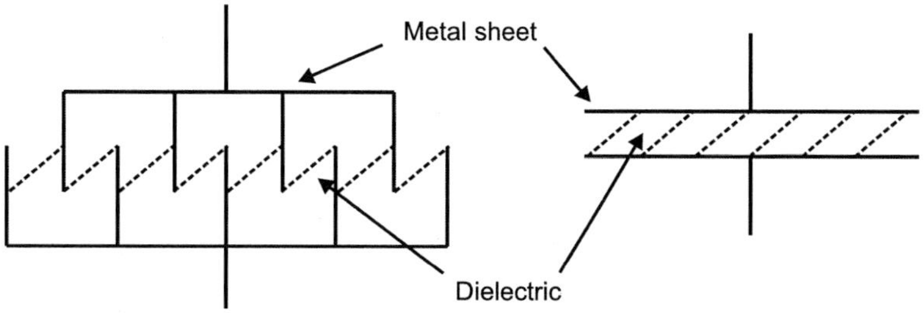

(a) Capacitor with large capacity (b) Capacitor with small capacity

Fig. 12.1: Structure of capacitor

Types

Capacitors are classified as:

- *Fixed capacitor:* Capacity is fixed (Fig. 12.2).
- *Variable capacitor:* Capacity can be varied.

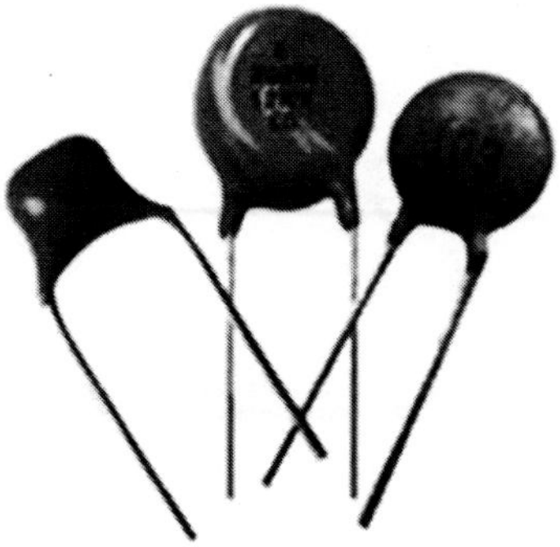

Fig. 12.2: A capacitor

Capacitor is also classified as:

- *Non-polarized:* It can be connected either way in a circuit. Ceramic, mica and some electrolytic capacitors are non-polarized. It is also called as bipolar capacitors.
- *Polarized:* It is a type of capacitor that has implicit polarity. It can only be connected one way in a circuit (Fig. 12.3)..

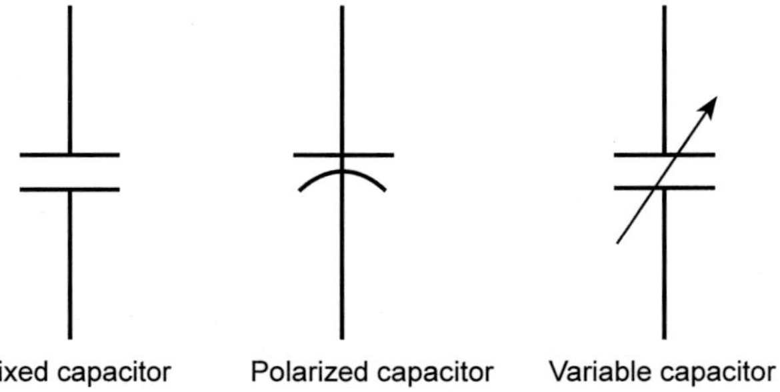

Fig. 12.3: Pictorial representation of a capacitor

Basic Types are as follows:

- *Ceramic capacitor:* In this, there is a dielectric medium with metal sheet.
- *Film capacitor:* In this, two metal sheets separated by a plastic film.
- Electrolytic capacitor metal anode and its oxidized material, e.g., Aluminium and Aluminium oxide.
- *Variable capacitor:* Capacitor can be varied by the knob.
- *Polystyrene capacitor:* Two sheets of aluminium foil separated by thin film.
- *Super capacitor:* It, initially, discharge a large amount of current.

Factors which determines the capacity:

Capacity tells ability to hold electric charge which is determined by:

- Surface area of plate.
- Material of plate.
- Width of the dielectric or space: If the width is very narrow there is more capacity.
- Dielectric medium: If it is a material than air it hold more charge compared to air (Fig. 12.4).
- No of plates connected in parallel.

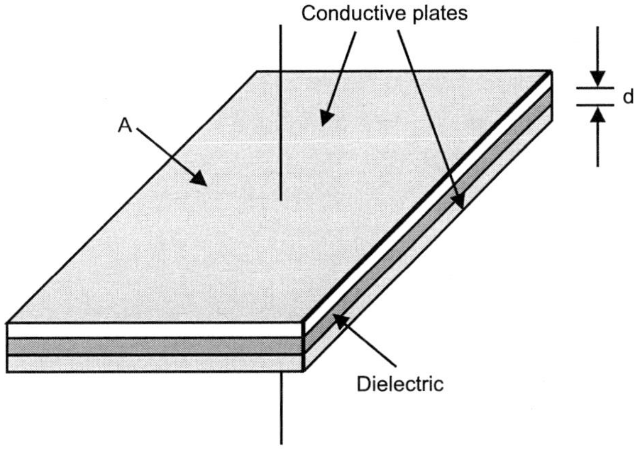

Fig. 12.4: Factors which determines the capacity

WORKING OF THE CAPACITOR

Charging a Condenser

A condenser can be charged directly by connecting the two plates to the opposite poles of a source of supply. The electrons pass from negative pole to one plate which becomes negatively charged and from the other plate to the positive and leaving this plate with positively charged. Initially when the intensity of the current is great the charging will be rapidly. The resulting charge on the plate opposes the current flow then the intensity becomes less and the rate of charging is slow. When a condenser is charged it can be disconnected from the source of supply and the charge is retained.

Discharge of a Condenser

When a circuit is completed between the plates of a charged condenser the electrons flow from negative to positive plate until the charge is neutralized. Initially, the intensity of the current is great, the condenser will discharge rapidly. In the later stage, condenser will discharge slowly.

Uses of Capacitor

1. *Smoothing circuit:* A smoothing circuit consists of inductor (L) and two capacitors (C_1 and C_2) which prevent the rapid rise of the current by inductor and prevent rapid fall of current by capacitor (Fig. 12.5).

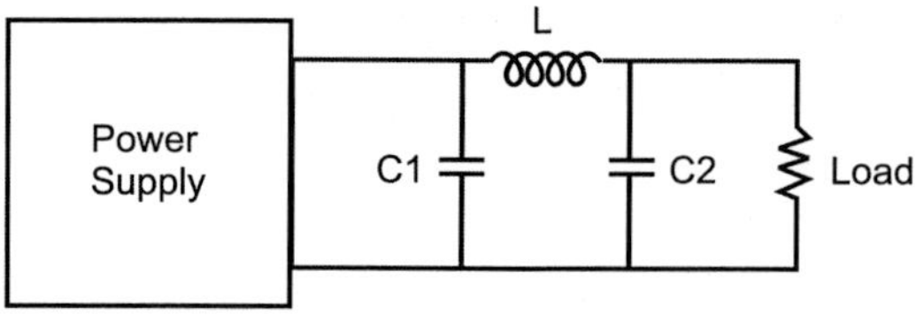

Fig. 12.5: Smoothing circuit

2. To make the current more comfortable for the patient, i.e., reduced sensory stimulation by producing damped oscillation.
3. *Used in tuning in short wave diathermy:* Varying the capacitance allows a circuit to be tuned to match the frequency of another oscillating circuit, thereby facilitating maximum transfer of energy between the two circuits.
4. Control timing in the stimulator (Fig. 12.6).

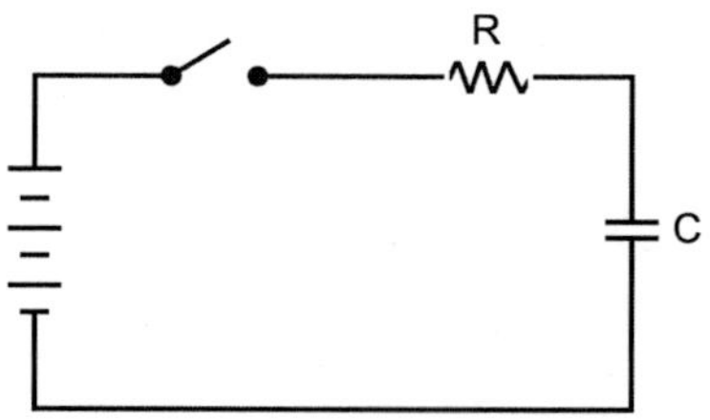

Fig. 12.6: The R C timing circuit

5. Capacitor is used along with triode valve and inductor to produced short wave which is of undamped oscillations.
6. Capacitors are also used for the surging of current.

13

Transformer

DEFINITION

It is a device which is used to alter the voltage of AC or to render a current earth free.

Principle

Electromagnetic induction.

Construction

Transformer consists of two coils of insulated wire (primary and secondary) and wind around a laminated soft iron frame. The frame is often rectangular in shape. The coil may wind up on the opposite side of the bars of frame (Fig. 13.1A) or one on top of the other on a central bar (Fig. 13.1B).

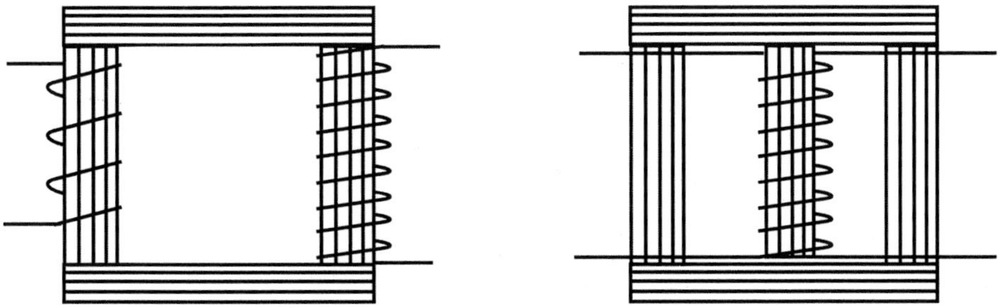

A B

Fig. 13.1A and B: Construction of a transformer

Working

An alternating current is passed through primary coil this sets up a varying magnetic field which cuts the secondary coil. By electromagnetic induction EMF is induced in the secondary circuit.

Functions

- To alter the voltage of a alternating current:
  - To bring down the voltage
  - To increase voltage.
- To render a current earth free.

If accidental connection is made between wire and earth, current will flow along it. If this connection is made by a person, they will receive a shock as a current flow through them to the earth. The static transformer reduces this danger by using electromagnetic induction to transfer electrical energy into secondary coil where earth place no path in the circuit.

Types of Transformer

- Static/even ratio
- Step down transformer
- Step up transformer
- Variable transformer
- Autotransformer.

Static transformer (isolation transformer or insulating transformer or even ratio transformer):

- Both primary and secondary coil have same number of turns (Fig. 13.2).
- Voltage will be same.
- Purpose: To reduce a current earth free circuit.

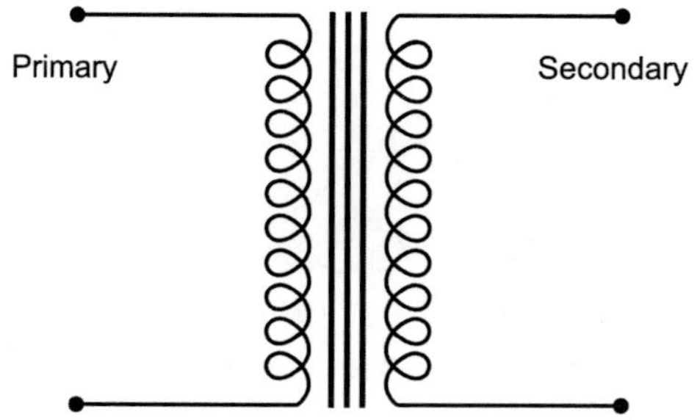

Fig. 13.2: Static transformer

Step Down Transformer

- The secondary coil has fewer turns than primary (Fig. 13.3).
- Voltage will be less than the primary.
- Purpose: To reduce voltage in the circuit.

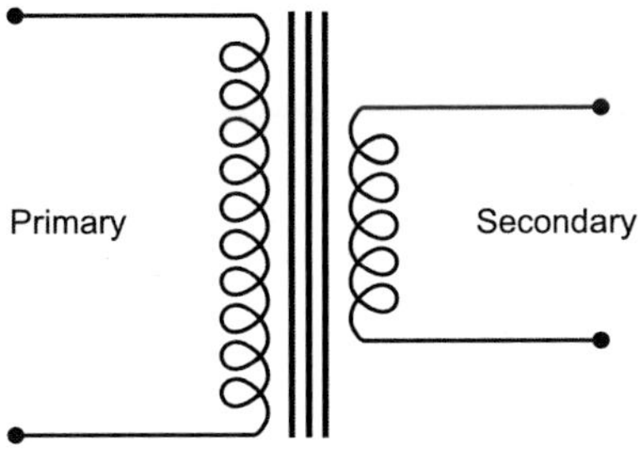

Fig. 13.3: Step down transformer

Step Up Transformer

- Secondary coil has more number of turns than primary (Fig. 13.4).
- Voltage will be more than the primary.
- Purpose: To increase the voltage in the circuit.

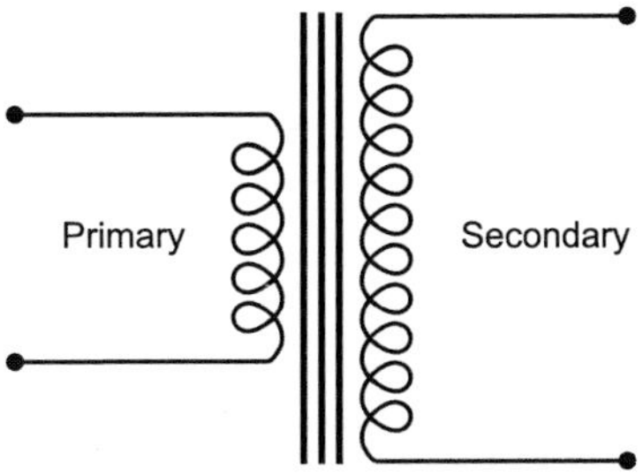

Fig. 13.4: Step up transformer

Variable Transformer

It consists of both primary and secondary coil.

Secondary coil has number of tapping taken from it and a movable contact can be placed on any of this by turning a switch. The effect of increasing the number of turns in the secondary coil relative to primary cause a step up voltage in the secondary coil (Fig. 13.5).

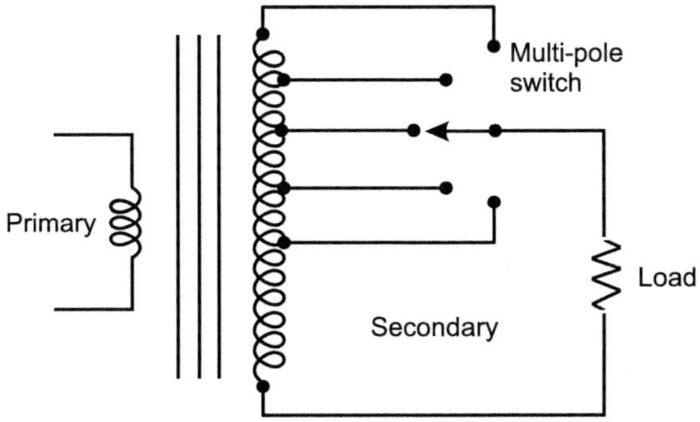

Fig. 13.5: Variable transformer

Auto Transformer

It is a single coil of wire with four contact points coming from it. It can work as both step up or step down transformer. For step up C and D will be primary and A and B will be secondary. For step down A and B is primary. C and D is secondary (Fig. 13.6).

Disadvantage: More chance of getting shock.

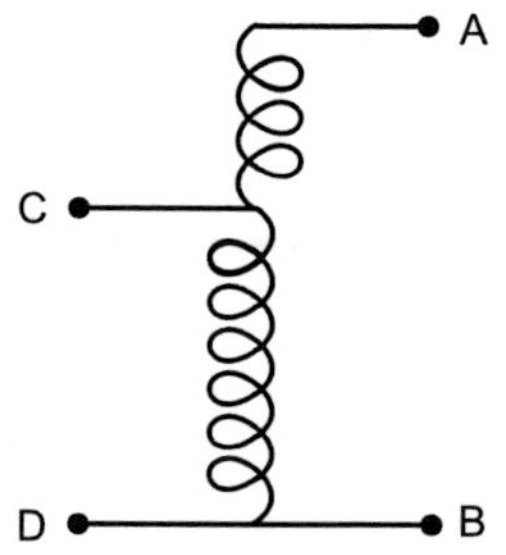

Fig. 13.6: Auto transformer

Application of transformer is physiotherapy

- Auto transformer will be used in the starter circuit of the UVR lamp and it is introduced into the circuit to strike the arc in the lamp.
- Variable transformer is used to adjust intensity in SWD and MWD.
- Step down transformer is used to produce DC, faradic, galvanic, TENS and sinusoidal current.
- Even ratio transformer are used for all the equipment to prevent the shock.

14

Valve

DEFINITION

It is a device which transmit current in one direction.

Principle

Thermionic emission: It is the emission of electrons from hot filament in vacuum.

TYPES

- Diode valve (Fig. 14.1A).
- Triode valve (Fig. 14.1B).

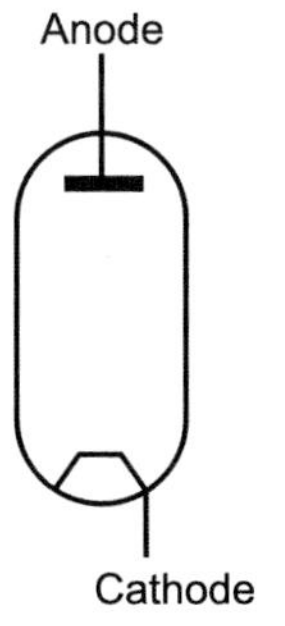

Fig. 14.1A: Diode value

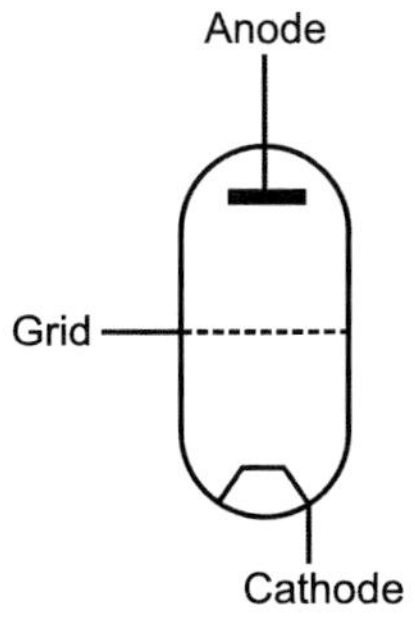

Fig. 14.1B: Triode valve

Diode Valve

Construction: A diode valve consists of a filament and a plate enclosed in an evacuated glass bulb (Fig. 14.1A).

Working: If potential difference is applied, the filament gets heated up and thermionic emission takes place. The electron moves towards anode (C to A) and the circuit is completed. If potential difference is reversed, heating does not take place and electrons will not move towards anode. Hence, current passes only in one direction (Fig.14.2).

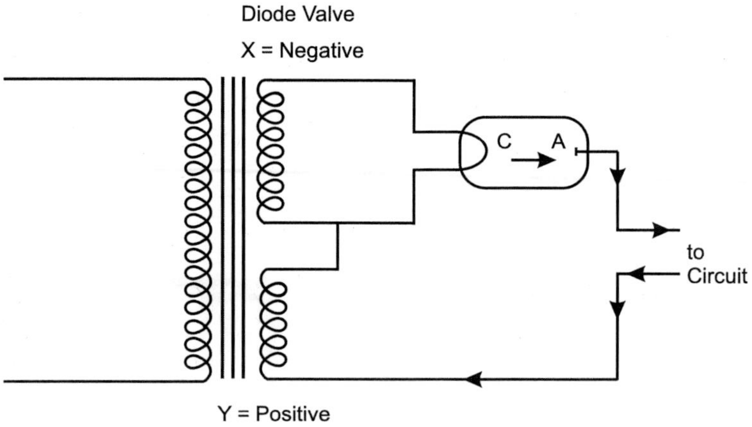

Fig. 14.2: Working of diode valve

Factors Determining the Intensity of Current

- Heating of the filament which results in more release of electrons.
- Increased potential difference between filament and the plate, results in more force of attraction for electron from the anode.

Triode Valve

Construction: Triode valve consists of three electrodes; Anode, Cathode and Grid. A grid can be connected to negative side or to the positive side (Fig. 14.3A).

Working: In addition to grid working is same as the diode valve (Fig. 14.3B).

Function of the Grid

If grid is positive, it attracts the electrons hence, there is more current flow.

If grid is negatively charged, it repels the electrons hence, there is no current flow.

If grid is neutral, it will act as same as that of diode valve.

Uses of Valves

- In half-wave rectification.
- In full-wave rectification.
- For production of short-wave.

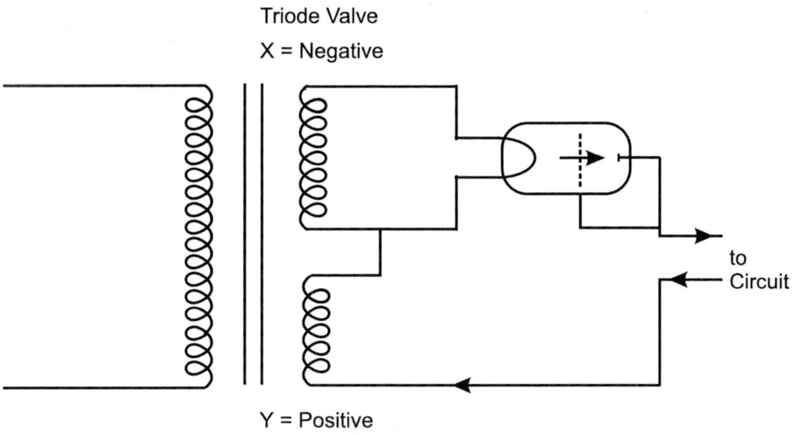

(A) When grid is connected to positive

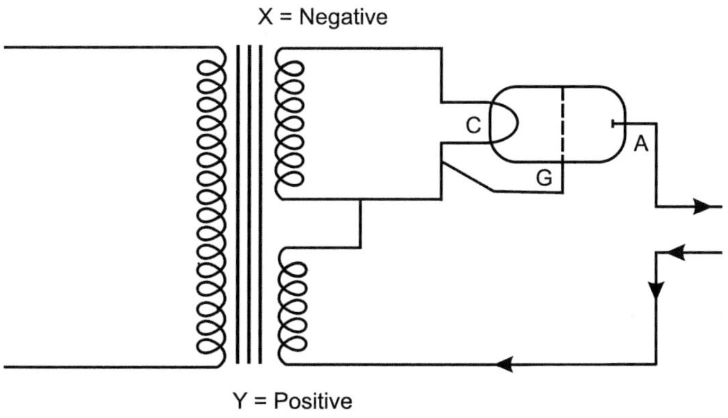

(B) When grid is connected to negative

Fig. 14.3: Construction of triode valve

15

Choke Coil

INTRODUCTION

The name comes from 'choking' which means blocking high frequencies while passing low frequencies. It is a functional name; the name 'choke' is used if an inductor is used for blocking or decoupling higher frequencies, but is simply called an 'inductor' if used in electronic filters or tuned circuits. In a circuit, choke coil is included in order to produce a self-induced EMF.

Definition

A choke is an inductor used to block higher-frequency alternating current (AC) in an electrical circuit, while passing lower-frequency or direct current (DC). These coils are used in a number of electrical devices. When used as part of a radio's circuitry, it falls into one of two frequency classes: audio or radio. Those used in circuits with higher frequencies use different core materials than those used in lower frequency circuits.

Apparatus

A choke usually consists of a coil of insulated wire wound on a magnetic core, although some consist of a donut-shaped 'bead' of ferrite material strung on a wire (Fig. 15.1). The choke's impedance increases with frequency. Its low electrical resistance passes both AC and DC with little power loss, but it can limit the amount of AC due to its reactance.

Working

The choke coil works because it acts as an inductor. When the current passing through changes, as AC currents does, it typically creates a magnetic field in the coil that works against that current. This property, known as inductance, blocks most of the AC current from passing through. As a result, currents that do not change, such as, DC currents, can continue through while those that do are blocked by the very magnetic field they created.

Types and Construction

Low-frequency Choke Coil

This consists of many turns of insulated wire wound on a laminated soft iron frame usually on the central bar of a rectangular frame. When a current which is varying in intensity is passed through the coil, magnetic lines of force are set up which cut the turns of wire and induce EMF's in them. There are many turns of wire so the coil has a considerable inductance and self-induced EMF produced will be large.

High-frequency Choke Coil

A high-frequency current varies very rapidly in intensity so tends to produce a considerable self-induced EMF. Because of this phenomenon, a high-frequency choke coil will not have more number of turns and coils may not be winded on iron core. Usually in a high-frequency coil insulated wire are wound on some non-conducting material.

Audio Frequency Chokes

Audio frequency chokes (AFC) usually have ferromagnetic cores to increase their inductance. They are often constructed similarly to transformers, with laminated iron cores and an air gap. A major use in the past was in power rectifiers and direct current motor controllers to produce direct current (DC), where they were used in conjunction with large electrolytic capacitors to remove the voltage ripple (AC) at the output DC.

Radiofrequency Chokes

Radio frequency chokes (RFC) often have iron powder or ferrite cores. They are often wound in complex patterns (basket winding) to reduce self-capacitance and proximity effect losses.

Common Mode Chokes

Common mode chokes, where two coils are wound on a single core, are useful for prevention of electromagnetic interference (EMI) and radiofrequency interference (RFI) from power supply lines and for prevention of malfunctioning of electronic equipment.

Uses of Choke Coil in Physiotherapy

It is included in the smoothing circuit. The self-induced EMF which is set up when a varying current is passed through a choke coil, it retards the rise of current to maximum and prolongs the current flow when the intensity is falling. This tends to even out the variations in the intensity of the current.

When a high-frequency current is passed through a choke coil the inductive reactance created will impede the flow of such current. So, choke coil is included in the circuit to allow low-frequency current and prevent high-frequency current.

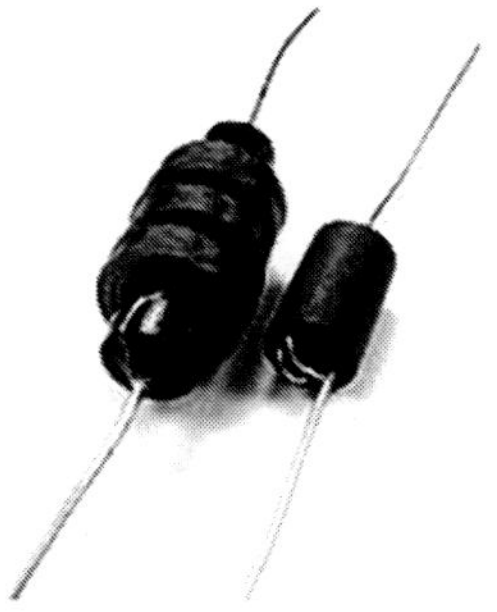

Fig. 15.1: A choke coil

16

Rectifying Devices

SEMICONDUCTORS

Definition

The materials that are neither conductor nor insulator with energy gap of about 1 eV (electron volt) are called semiconductors. Most common type of semiconductors is germanium (Ge) and silicon (Si), because of their property to withstand high temperature.

Principle

A conductor of electricity is a material, usually a metal, in which are free electrons which readily move to constitute an electric current. An insulator is a material in which the electrons are firmly held, either by their central nuclei or by forming bonds with other atoms to build up the crystalline structure, so that they are not free to move. At room temperature resistivity of semiconductor is in between insulators and conductors. Semiconductors show negative temperature coefficient of resistivity that means its resistance decreases with increase in temperature. Both Si and Ge are elements of IV group, i.e., both elements have 4 valence electrons. Both form the covalent bond with the neighboring atom. At absolute zero temperature both behave as insulator, i.e., the valence band is full while conduction band is empty but as the temperature is raised more and more, thermal agitation of the molecules can free some of the electrons from their bonds. The covalent bonds break and electrons are set free, jump to their conduction band and thus, capable of transmitting current.

Types

Semiconductors are divided into intrinsic and extrinsic semiconductors. Semiconductor in its pure form is called as intrinsic semiconductors whereas impure semiconductors are called extrinsic semiconductors. In pure semiconductor number of electrons (n) is equal to number of holes (p) and thus, conductivity is very low as valence electrons are covalent bonded. Extrinsic semiconductor is formed by adding a small amount of impurity. Depending on the type of impurity added we have two types of semiconductors: N-type and P-type semiconductors. In 100 million parts of semiconductor, one part of impurity is added.

N-type Semiconductor

In this type of semiconductor, majority carriers are electrons and minority carriers are holes. N-type semiconductor is formed by adding pentavalent (five valence electrons) impurity in pure semiconductor crystal, e.g., P, As, Sb. Four of the five valence electron of pentavalent impurity forms covalent bond with Si atom and the remaining electron is free to move anywhere within the crystal. Pentavalent impurity donates electron to Si that's why N-type impurity atoms are known as donor atoms. This enhances the conductivity of pure Si.

P-type Semiconductor

In this type of semiconductor, majority carriers are holes and minority carriers are electrons. P-type semiconductor is formed by adding trivalent (three valence electrons) impurity in pure semiconductor crystal, e.g., B, Al, Ba. Three of the four valence electron of tetravalent impurity forms covalent bond with Si atom. This leaves an empty space which is referred to as hole. When temperature is raised electron from another covalent bond jumps to fill this empty space. This leaves a hole behind. In this way conduction takes place. P-type impurity accepts electron and is called acceptor atom.

Contact between Semiconductors: When an n-type semiconductor, which has free electrons, is placed in contact with a p-type semiconductor, which has positive holes, electrons move from the former to occupy holes in the latter, while positive holes move in the reverse direction. Both were originally electrically neutral, so the transfer of electrons sets up a P.D. at the junction, the p-type semiconductor a negative charge. The transfer of electrons continues until a certain P.D. is established, then this prevents any further electron movement.

Conduction Across Semiconductor Junction

When the semiconductors are connected to a source of EMF, the P.D. at their junction affects the flow of current. If the n-type semiconductor is made more negative than the equilibrium value and the p-type more positive, electrons lost from the former are replaced from the supply, while excess electrons are withdrawn from the latter to the supply. The P.D. at the junction is reduced, electrons are able to pass from the n-type to the p-type semiconductor and current flows in the circuit. If, however, the p-type semiconductor is made negative relative to the n-type, the P.D. at the junction opposes the electron movement and no current can flow until the applied P.D. reaches a certain critical valve. Therefore, current can pass more easily in one direction than in the other, and the device constitutes a semiconductor diode.

Metal Rectifiers

A metal rectifier works on the same principle as the semiconductor diode, and one type consists of a copper disc coated on one surface with copper oxide. Copper oxide is a p-type semiconductor and copper, being a metal, has free electrons, and so acts like an n-type semiconductor. Thus, when the two materials are in contact a P.D. is set up at their junction. When the rectifier is connected into a circuit with the copper negative relative to the copper oxide, current passes much more easily than when the polarity is reversed. In the latter case, no current flows until the EMF exceeds 8 volts. A series of discs can be used to rectify larger voltages, but must be separated from each other by suitable materials; otherwise the P.D.s developed at the contacts would cancel each other out.

The construction and symbol for the rectifiers are shown. In the symbol (Fig. 16.1), the arrow head represents the copper, i.e., shows the direction of electron flow.

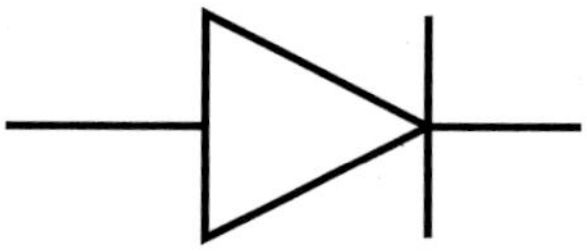

Fig. 16.1: Symbol of a metal rectifier

TRANSISTORS

A transistor consists of two thick layers of one type of semiconductor, termed the emitter and the collector, separated by a thin layer of the other type of semiconductor, termed the base. In a p-n-p transistor the emitter and the collector are of p-type, the base of n-type semiconductor, while in the n-p-n transistor the position of the materials is reversed.

Fig. 16.2: Position of materials in PNP and NPN transistor

Working of NPN Transistor

As soon as contact is made between the materials, P.D. is developed at their junctions. In an n-p-n transistor the emitter and the collector are of n-type semiconductor so both become positive relative to the p-type base (Fig. 16.3).

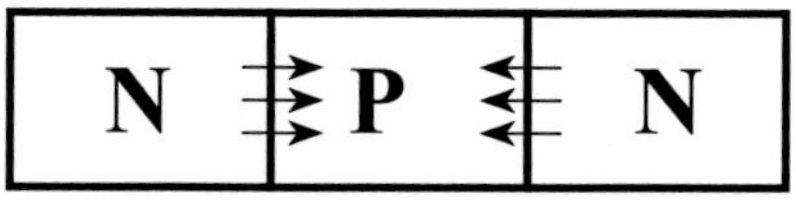

Fig. 16.3: NPN transistor at rest

If the device is then connected to a source of EMF with the emitter negative and the collector positive, no current flows unless the EMF exceeds the critical value. Electrons could cross the emitter-base junction but are unable to pass from the base to the collector, as the movement is opposed by the junction P.D. (Fig 16.4).

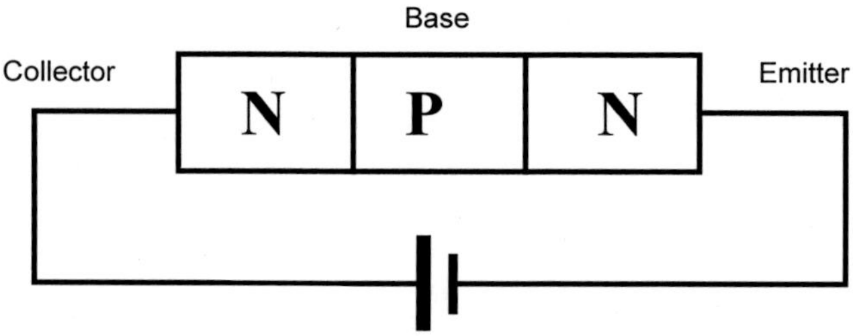

Fig. 16.4: NPN transistor connected to a source of EMF

When, however, a second source of EMF is connected to the base and the emitter, with the base positive relative to the emitter the transistor becomes capable of transmitting current. Electrons can cross from the negative n-type emitter to the positive p-type base, so current flows in this emitter-base circuit. In this circuit, there is a thick layer of n-type semiconductor, a thin layer of the p-type, so the current consists largely of a movement of electrons, and electrons from the emitter soon pass into the base. The base now has an adequate supply of electrons, and as it is very thin these come close to the base-collector junction and are attached into the collector to replace those that had migrated into the base. This reduces the barrier effect at the base-collector junction and current flows across the transistor (Fig. 16.5).

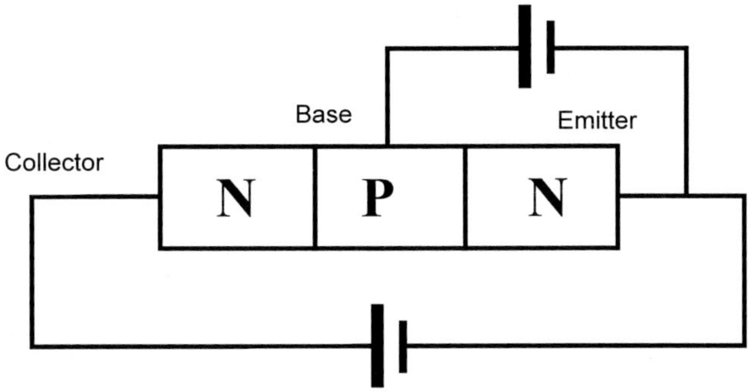

Fig. 16.5: Transistor connected to a second source

Thus, a current fed into the base renders the transistor capable of conducting current, and small variations in this base current produce much greater variations in the current flowing across the transistor. In this respect, the current fed into the base of a transistor has an effect comparable to that of a positive charge applied to the grid of a triode valve.

Figure 16.6 which is given below is the symbol of PNP and NPN transistor. Commercially available transistors is shown in Figure 16.7.

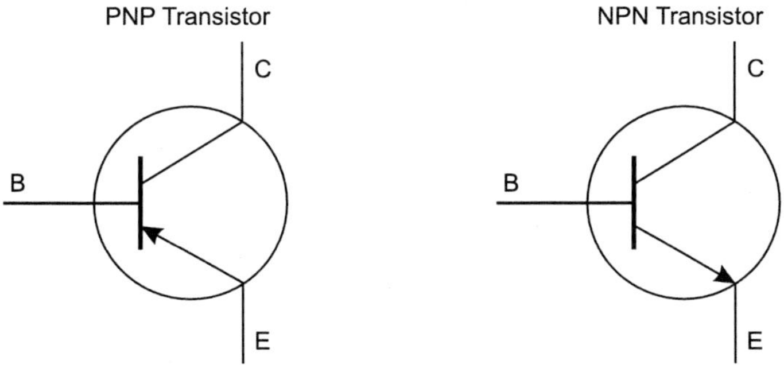

Fig. 16.6: Symbolic representation of PNP and NPN transistor

Uses of transistor: It can act as switch or as an amplifier. Transistors are used in preference to valves in much modern electrical equipment. They have the advantages of durability, long life and low power consumption, and do not require a heating circuit. The power output is, however, limited, so while they are suitable for use in electronic stimulators they are not as yet generally used to replace the valves of short-wave diathermy machines.

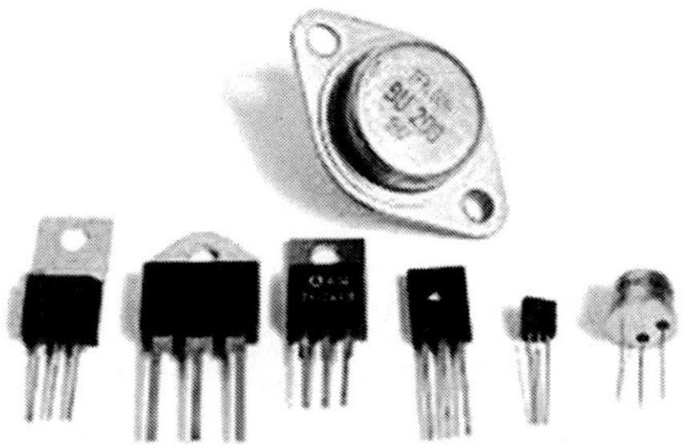

Fig. 16.7: Commercially available transistors

TRANSDUCER

Definition

A transducer is a device that converts one form of energy to another. Transducer is the other term, i.e., sometimes interchangeably used instead of the term sensor, although there are subtle differences. The process of converting one form of energy to another is known as transduction.

Types of Transducer

Active: Active sensors require an external power sources to operate, which is called an excitation signal. The signal is modulated by the sensor to produce the output signal. For example, a thermistor does not generate any electric signal, but by passing electric current through it, its resistance can be measured by detecting variations in current and/or voltage across the thermistor.

Passive: Passive sensors generate electric signals in response to an external stimulus without the need of an additional energy source. Such examples are a thermocouple, photodiode, and a piezoelectric sensor.

Sensors: A sensor is a device that receives and responds to a signal or stimulus.

Actuators: An actuator is a device, i.e., responsible for moving or controlling a mechanism or system. It is operated by a source of energy, which can be mechanical force, electrical current, hydraulic fluid pressure, or pneumatic pressure, and converts that energy into motion. An actuator is the mechanism by which a control system acts upon an environment. The control system can be simple (a fixed mechanical or electronic system), software-based (e.g., a printer driver, robot control system), a human, or any other input.

Bidirectional: Bidirectional transducers convert physical phenomena to electrical signals and also convert electrical signals into physical phenomena. Examples of inherently bidirectional transducers are antennae, which can convert conducted electrical signals to or from propagating electromagnetic waves, and voice coils, which convert electrical signals into sound (when used in a loudspeaker) or sound into electrical signals (when used in a microphone). Likewise, DC electric motors may be used to generate electrical power if the motor shaft is turned by an external torque.

Applications

- Electromagnetic: Antenna, CD writer
- Electrochemical: pH probe

- Electromechanical: Pressure sensor
- Electroacoustic: Loud speaker, Ultrasound head
- Electro-optical: Laser diode
- Electrostatic: Electrometer
- Thermoelectric: Thermistor
- Radioacoustic: Transmitter.

AMPLIFIER

Definition

An amplifier is an electronic device that can increase the power of a signal. An amplifier functions by taking power from a power supply and controlling the output to match the input signal shape but with a larger amplitude. In this sense, an amplifier modulates the output of the power supply based upon the properties of the input signal. An amplifier is effectively the opposite of an attenuator: while an amplifier provides gain, an attenuator provides loss.

The actual amplifier component may be a Transistor or Vacuum tube or Magnetic amplifier.

Classification

Amplifiers can be categorized in different ways. One is by the frequency of the electronic signal being amplified; audio amplifiers amplify signals in the audio (sound) range of less than 20 kHz, RF amplifiers amplify frequencies in the radio frequency range between 20 kHz and 300 GHz. Another is which quantity, voltage or current is being amplified; amplifiers can be divided into Voltage Amplifiers, current amplifiers, Trans-conductance amplifiers, and Trans-resistance amplifiers (Table 16.1). LASER can be considered as light amplifier. Amplifier is incorporated in nerve conduction studies and EMG.

Table 16.1: Classification of electronic amplifier

Input	*Output*	*Dependent source*	*Amplifier type*	*Gain units*
I	I	Current controlled current source CCCS	Current amplifier	Unit less
I	V	Current controlled voltage source CCVS	Trans resistance amplifier	Ohm
V	I	Voltage controlled current source VCCS	Trans conductance amplifier	Siemens
V	V	Voltage controlled voltage source VCVS	Voltage amplifier	Unit less

OSCILLATOR CIRCUIT

Introduction

An oscillator circuit produces a periodic, oscillating electronic signal, often a sine wave or a square wave.

Components

An LC circuit, also called a resonant circuit, tank circuit, or tuned circuit, is an electric circuit consisting of an inductor, represented by the letter L, and a capacitor, represented by the letter C, connected together. The circuit can act as an electrical resonator, an electrical analog of a tuning fork, storing energy oscillating at the circuit's resonant frequency. It can be a series resonant circuit or parallel resonant circuit. In a parallel circuit both inductor and capacitor are connected in parallel whereas they are connected one after another (Fig. 16.8).

Working

If the charged capacitor is discharged through a circuit of low ohmic resistance which includes an inductance, electrons flow forward then back between the plates in an oscillating manner. The reason for this sequence of events is that as current flows through the inductance, self-induced EMF's are produced. These back EMF impede electron flow, but when both plates reach the same potential the forward EMF causes an electron flow onto one plate with the result that it becomes negatively charged. This sequence continues as a series of damped oscillations (Fig. 16.9) until all the energy in the system is exhausted. The frequency of the current thus, obtained is calculated below:

$F = 1/2\pi\sqrt{LC}$

Where f = frequency, C = capacity and L = inductance

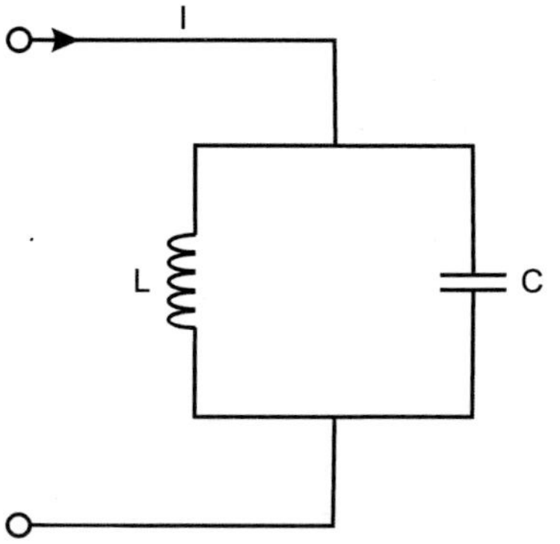

Fig. 16.8: LC circuit in parallel

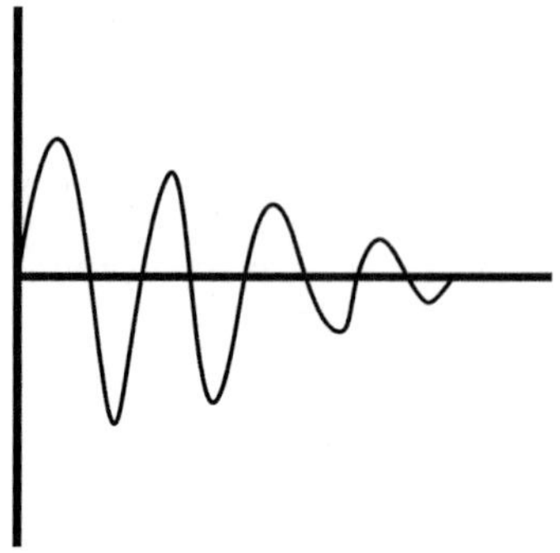

Fig. 16.9: Damped oscillations

Uses

LC circuit has many important applications in signal processing and communications systems, such as in tuning current magnification, voltage magnification and RF amplifier. They are also used in induction heating. In physiotherapy, the oscillator circuit forms the basis of machine, such as, the short wave diathermy and ultrasonic apparatus which require a high-frequency current to operate.

RECTIFIER

Definition

Rectifier is a device which converts AC to DC. Two types of rectifier are used in the physiotherapy. They are Thermionic valve or diode valve and Metal rectifier.

Types of Rectification

- Half wave rectification: The current passes only in one direction and the flow is blocked during alternate half cycle of AC (Fig. 16.10).
- Full wave rectification: The current passes in one direction and the alternate half cycle is reversed so that a continuous current is produced.

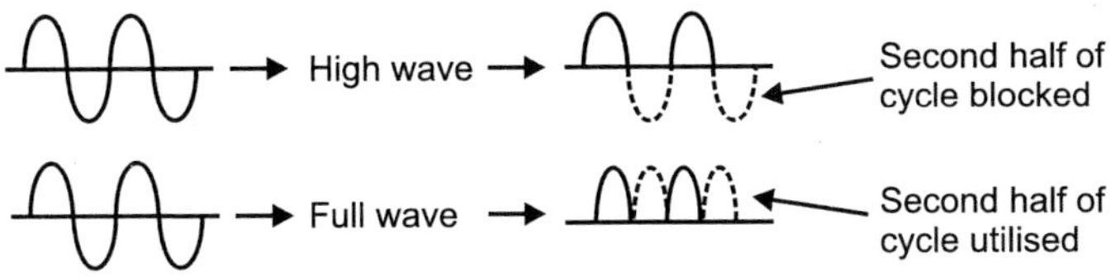

Fig. 16.10: Half wave and full wave rectification

Methods to Produce Half Wave Rectification

With the help of diode valve:

Working: If potential difference is applied (when X = negative), the filament gets heated up and thermionic emission takes place. The electron moves towards anode and the circuit is completed. If potential difference is reversed (when X = positive), heating does not take place and electrons will not move towards anode. Hence, current passes only in one direction (Fig. 16.11).

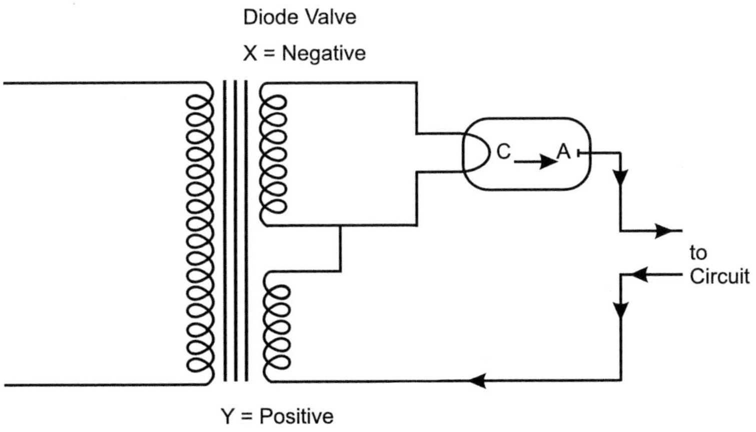

Fig. 16.11: Half wave rectification with the help of diode valve

With the help of metal rectifier:

When X is negative, Copper releases the electron which moves towards copper oxide. Current goes through circuit and reaches the Y. When X is positive, Copper will not release the electron. So, there is no current flow. Hence current passes only in one direction (Fig. 16.12).

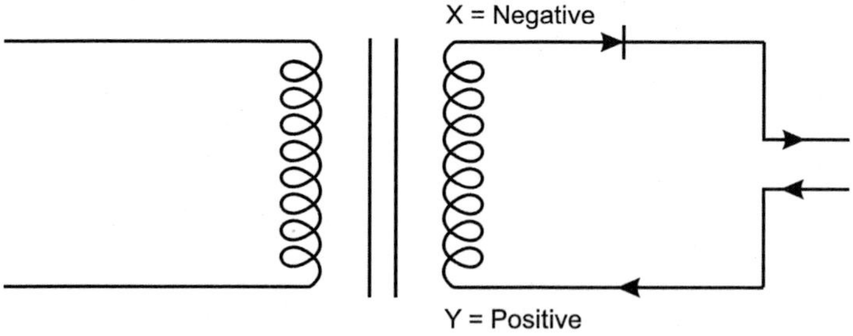

Fig. 16.12: Half wave rectification with metal rectifier

Methods of Producing Full Wave Rectification

Voltage halving circuit with the help of rectifier:

Only half of the secondary coil of the transformers is used during each half of AC so the EMF supplied to the patient circuit is always half of which is used in primary coil.

When X is negative, it cannot pass through rectifier A. But, Z is negative compared to Y. So current passes through patient circuit. It cannot cross rectifier A because X is negative. It crosses rectifier B and reaches Y thus completing the circuit. Finally, the first half rectification is done (Fig. 16.13A).

When X is positive and Y is negative, it cannot cross rectifier B. But, Z is more negative compared to X. So, current passes through patient circuit. It passes through rectifier A and reaches X. Thus, next half rectification is also done (Fig. 16.13B).

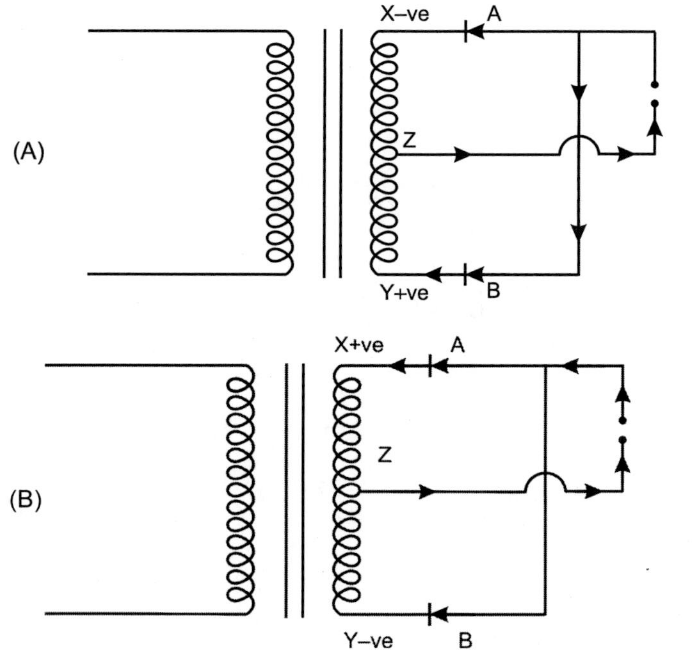

Fig. 16.13: Full wave rectification with rectifiers

Voltage Halving Circuit with the Help of Diode Valve

Here, the diode valve with two anodal plates is used.

When X is negative, there is no current flow. But, Z is more negative compared to Y so current flows through Z. The current reaches the filament circuit and filament is heated. Electron is released and move towards A1 and A2, A1 get attracted and A2 gets repelled. So, it passes through A1and reaches to Y. Thus, the initial half of rectification is done (Fig. 16.14A).

When Y is negative, there is no current flow. But, Z is more negative compared to Y, so current flows through Z. The current reaches filament circuit and filament is heated. Electron is released and move towards A1 and A2, A1 get repelled and A2 gets attracted. So, it passes through A2 and reaches to X. Thus, next half rectification is done (Fig. 16.14B).

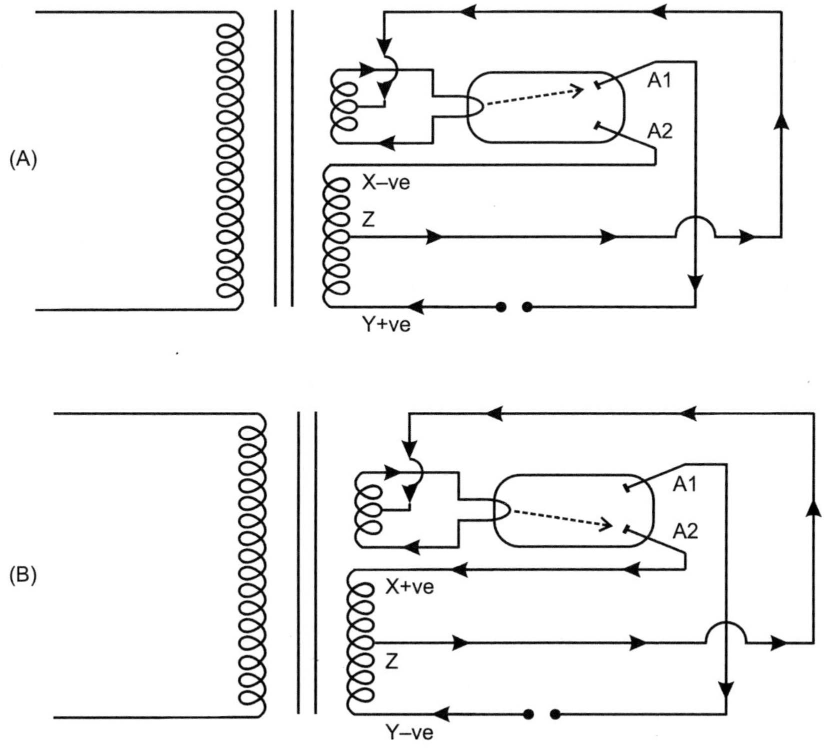

Fig. 16.14: Full wave rectification with diode valve

Full Voltage Circuit with Wheatstone Bridge or Westinghouse Bridge

Construction

Four rectifiers are used to make diamond arrangement. The input wires are connected to opposite corners and output is taken from another two corners. Two rectifiers, A and B are directed towards one output wire and the other two rectifiers, C and D away from 2nd output wire.

Working

When X is negative: It cannot cross D but can cross A. It reaches patient circuit. It returns back to Y through C. It cannot cross through B and D. Thus, half wave rectification is done (Fig. 16.15A).

When Y is negative: It cannot cross C but crosses B. It reaches patient circuit. It returns back to X through D. It cannot cross A and C. Thus, another half-rectification is done (Fig. 16.15B).

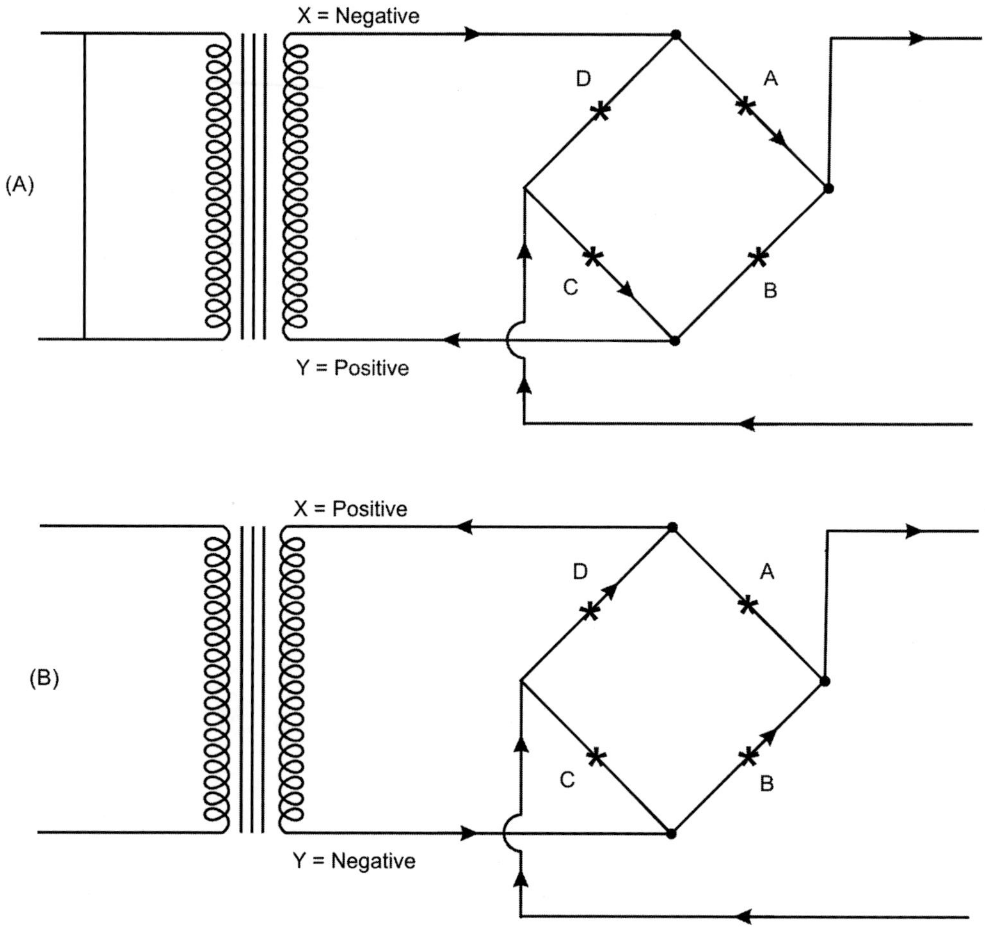

Fig. 16.15: Full wave rectification with Wheatstone bridge

17

Display Devices and Indicators

INTRODUCTION

A **display device** is an output device for presentation of information in visual or tactile form (the latter used, e.g., in tactile electronic displays for blind people). The display system is the final link between the measuring process and the user. In the instruments, these devices are used to provide instantaneous but non-permanent communication of information between a process or system and a human observer.

Commonly used display techniques and its mechanism:

- **Moving pointer:** Mechanical or electromechanical movement of a pointer over a fixed scale.
- **Moving scale or electromechanical movement of a scale:** The indication given by position of scale with respect to fixed pointer.
- **Bar graph:** Indication given by height or length of vertical or horizontal column.
- **Light emitting diodes:** Light output provided by recombination electroluminescence in a forward biased semiconductor diode.
- **Liquid crystal display:** The modulation of intensity of transmitted reflected light by the application of an electric field to a liquid crystal cell.
- **CRT displays:** Conversion into light of the energy of scanning electron beam by phosphor.

Classification of display systems:

1. On methods of conversion of electrical data into visible light:
   (a) Active display: Cathode ray tube, light emitting diode.
   (b) Passive display: light controller, electrophoretic image display.
2. On the applications:
   (a) Analog display: Cathode ray tube, bar graph display.
   (b) Digital display: Nixie tube, Alphanumeric, LEDs.

3. According to the display size and physical dimension:
   (a) Symbolic displays: Nixie tube, Alphanumeric, LEDs.
   (b) Console displays: CRTs, LEDs, etc.
   (c) Large screen display: Enlarged projection system.
4. According to the display format:
   (a) Direct view type or planar type: Segmental dot-matrix; CRT.
   (b) Stacked electrode or nonplanar type: Nixie.
5. In terms of resolution and legibility of characters:
   (a) Simple single-element indicators.
   (b) Multi-element displays.

In Physiotherapy equipments, data can be presented to the observer in either an analog or digital form. Analog displays use a needle and calibrated scale to indicate values. They have a pointer which moves over a graduated scale. In this display, values are difficult to read. Digital displays show the measured value as digits. They are more accurate than analog, easier to use, can display even small values.

18

Production of An EMF by Chemical Action

DEFINITION

In current electricity, cell means an electrochemical cell. Cell is a device by which chemical energy is converted into electrical energy.

Principles of Cells

An EMF is produced by chemical action in a cell. The cell consists of two dissimilar metals immersed in an electrolyte and the principle underlying its action is based on the behavior of a metal immersed in a solution. Metals at different points in the electrochemical series are chosen, one above and the other below hydrogen. When they are immersed in the electrolyte ions pass from one metal into the solution and this electrode becomes negatively charged. Ions from the solution are deposited on the other electrode which consequently acquires a positive charge. Thus, a P.D. is set up between the metals. The ionic movement continues only until a certain P.D. is established between each metal and the solution. The voltage available from the cell is the sum of these potential differences and the EMF produced, therefore, depends on the position of the metals in the electrochemical series and on the electrolyte used. A particular combination of materials always provides the same EMF.

On completion of a pathway between the electrodes, outside the cell, electrons pass through this external circuit from the negative to the positive electrode. The flow of electrons tends to reduce the charge on both electrodes, but as this occurs the movement of ions within the cell recommences, maintaining the charge on the electrodes and so the P.D. between them. The negative potential of one metal and the positive potential of the other remain constant throughout, so the current obtained is direct and unvarying. The current flow is impeded not only by the resistance of the external circuit but also within the cell itself, where there is some impedance to the movement of ions. The latter is referred to as the internal resistance of the cell.

Types

Electrochemical cells are of two types:

1. The primary cells.
2. The secondary cells.

The primary cells are those in which electrical energy is produced due to chemical energy. The chemical reaction in the primary cell is irreversible. The examples of primary cells are Voltaic cell, Daniel cell, Leclanche cell, Dry cell, etc.

The secondary cells are those in which the electrical energy is first stored up as the chemical energy. When current is required to drawn from the secondary cell, then the chemical energy is reconverted into the electrical energy. The chemical reaction in the secondary cell is reversible. The examples of secondary cells are Lead-acid accumulators, alkali accumulators or Edison cell. The initial cost of a primary cell is less as compared to the secondary cell. But, the running cost of a secondary cell is low as compared to the primary cell. The electrolytes, cathode and anode used and its uses are mentioned in Table 18.1.

Table 18.1: Characteristics of different types of cells

Type	*Cell*	*Electrolyte*	*Cathode*	*Anode*	*Uses*
Primary	Voltaic cell	Sulphuric acid	Zinc rod	Copper rod	–
Primary	Daniel cell	Copper sulphate	Porous pot containing amalgamated Zinc rod	Copper vessel	–
Primary	Leclanche cell	Ammonium chloride	Amalgamated Zinc rod	Porous pot with Carbon rod and Manganese dioxide and Charcoal powder	–
Primary	Dry cell	Ammonium chloride and Zinc chloride	Zinc vessel	Carbon rod and Manganese dioxide and charcoal in a muslin bag	Calculators torches
Primary	Mercury cell	Potassium hydroxide	Zinc	Steel	Long life hearing aids
Secondary	Lead acid accumulator	Sulphuric acid	Lead	Lead oxide	Car batteries
Secondary	Alkali accumulator or Edison cell or Nife cell	Potassium hydroxide and Lithium hydroxide	Steel grid, Iron hydrochloride and Mercury oxide	Perforated steel plate, Nickel hydrochloride and Nickel	Emergency light
Secondary	Nicad cell	Potassium hydroxide	Cadmium	Nickel oxide	Rechargeable batteries

Cells in Series and Parallel

If the cells are connected in series, the total EMF is the sum of the EMF's of the individual cells and the internal resistance of the battery is the sum of the internal resistances of the individual cells. If the cells are connected in parallel, the total EMF of the battery is the same as that of a single cell and the internal resistance is reduced to less than that of one cell. The choice of method of connecting the cells depends on the resistance of the external circuit. If the resistance is high, a large EMF is necessary to produce an appreciable intensity of current, and the cells are connected in series with each other to provide this. Even though the internal resistance is increased, it is negligible compared to resistance of circuit as a whole. Connection of cells in parallel has the additional advantage that they last longer than if a single cell is used. This arrangement makes internal resistance as low as possible.

19

Ionization

DEFINITION

When constant current is applied, there is two-way migration of ion which is called as ionization.

Types

- Medical ionization.
- Surgical ionization.

Medical ionization: It is also called as Iontophoresis.

Effects

- Increased vasodilatation.
- Anti-cholinergic effect: By the use of Glycoperronium bromide, Poldine methosulfate.
- Triple response: Histamine.
- Bactericidal effect: Potassium iodide, Zinc oxide.
- Anesthetic effect: Lidocaine.
- Analgesic effect: Salicylate, Lidocaine.
- Softening the scar: Sodium chloride.
- Muscle relaxant: Magnesium sulphate.
- Anti-inflammatory effect: Glucocorticoids, Dexamethasone, Hydrocortisone, Salicylate.
- Anti-allergic effect: Histamine.
- Anti-sudation effect (Antisweating): Tap water.

Surgical Ionization or Surgical Galvanism or Surgical Electrolysis

Destruction of unwanted tissue by DC is called as surgical ionisation or surgical electrolysis or electrochemical cauterisation. It is performed by plastic surgeons or dermatologist. Here cathode, which acts as an active electrode is in form of a needle and anode, is indifferent electrode. Half mA of direct current is applied for 1 minute. Skill is required for surgical galvanism. There are 10–20% chances of recurrence following this technique.

Indications

- Removal of unwanted hairs (Hypertrichosis).
- Removal of warts.
- Removal of carbuncle.
- Removal of boils.

20

Induction

DEFINITION

Production of electrical or magnetic property in one object by another without having contact in between them is called as induction.

Types

- Electrostatic induction (already discussed in earlier chapter).
- Electromagnetic induction.

Electromagnetic Induction

History: Discovered by Michael Faraday in 1831.

Definition: It is the production of electrical properties in one object which must be a conductor of electricity by magnetic line of force surrounding another object.

Factors responsible for Electromagnetic induction:

1. A conductor.
2. Magnetic line of force.
3. Relative movement of one and two.

Procedure

A coil of wire is connected to a milliampere ammeter to form a closed circuit.

Experiment 1: A bar magnet is introduced into the coil, deflection of the needle of the meter is observed in one direction (Fig. 20.1).

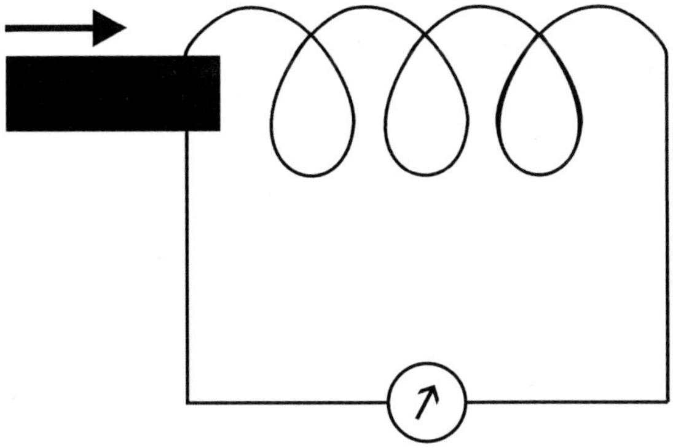

Fig. 20.1: Experiment 1

Experiment 2: When the bar magnet is remains stationary no deflection is observed in the meter (Fig. 20.2).

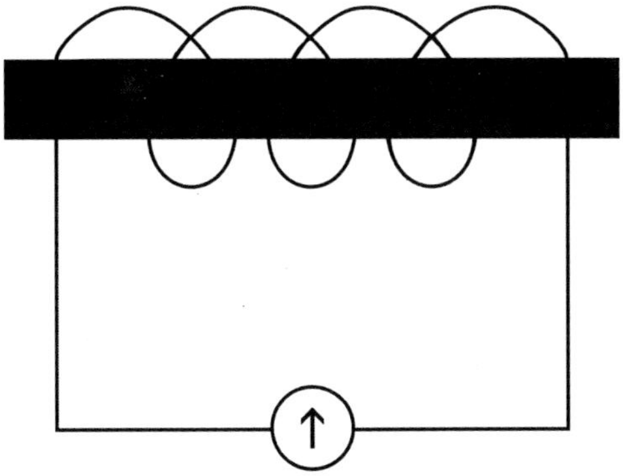

Fig. 20.2: Experiment 2

Experiment 3: A bar magnet is withdrawn from the coil the deflection is observed in the meter in opposite direction (Fig. 20.3).

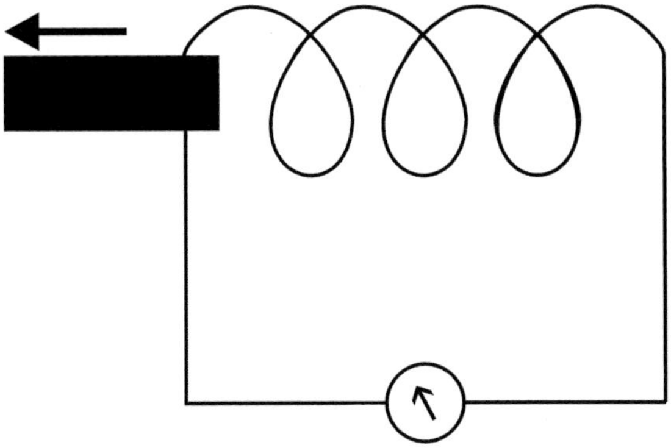

Fig. 20.3: Experiment 3

Laws Governing Electromagnetic Induction

Lenz's law: It states that, *the direction of induced EMF is such that it tends to oppose the force producing in it.*

Faraday's law of electromagnetic induction: It states that, *I, the strength of the induced EMF is proportional to rate of change of magnetic field. The strength of induced EMF is proportional to inductance of the conductor in which it is produced.*

The inductance is the ability of the conductor to have a current induced in it.

The factors which determine the inductance:

- Using many turns of the wire in the coil.
- Placing the turns close together.
- Winding the coil into soft iron core.

Types of induced EMF:

(a) Mutual induced EMF

When an EMF is induced in one conductor by the magnetic field set up by a varying current flowing in another conductor, the process is known as mutal induction.

(b) Self-induced EMF

When a current flow through a coil of wire itself, a induced EMF occur in a opposite direction and it opposes the main current, the process is known as self-induced EMF. It is also called as back EMF.

Eddy Current

If conductor is solid, the magnetic line of force passing through it will set up circular current called Eddy current. Eddy current is perpendicular to magnetic line of force. These currents tend to reduce magnetic effect of the current by setting up a magnetic field in opposition to the original one. Eddy current produce heating effect in accordance to Joules law. Eddy current is unwanted and can be prevented by laminating the conductor, i.e., cutting into the layer (split into strips) and insulating each layer from the other. These strips lie at right angles to the direction in which the currents would flow, electrons are unable to pass from one strip to next and so the currents are prevented. However, Eddy currents are useful in many ways. The principles of Eddy currents are used in induction cooker, induction motor, electromagnetic damping (to minimise deflection in galvanometer), speedometer and electromagnetic brakes. In Physiotherapy, SWD using inductotherapy method; Eddy current are used to produce heating effect in the tissue.

21

Main Supply

Production

Currents for main supply are produced by means of dynamos at the power stations. The essential principles of the dynamo is that an EMF is induced by the movement of a conductor and a magnetic field in relation to each other. Mechanical energy must be available to provide the movement. Water, oil, tidal waves, wind mill or steam are commonly used for the movement of dynamo. Either Coal fuel or nuclear energy is necessary to operate the steam engine.

Type of Current

With dynamo either A.C. or D.C. can be produced. For main distribution in earlier years D.C. was preferred. Now, it has been replaced by A.C.

Advantages of A.C. Compared to D.C. for Main Distribution

Distribution of A.C. has more advantages compared to D.C. in terms of production and distribution. Following are the advantages:

- The construction of the dynamo is such that a greater voltage can be produced with A.C. than with D.C.
- It is the possible to alter the voltage of A.C. with static transformers.
- The construction of much modern apparatus is such that it works only on an A.C. supply.
- Easier for long distance transmission.

When the current is to be carried for long distances, the EMF is stepped up to several thousand volts (above 13000 V) with a corresponding reduction in the intensity of current. This low intensity current can be carried by comparatively thin cables, which cost less than the thick ones required for currents of large intensities. Over long distances, there is a certain loss in voltage, but with the very high EMFs used this is only a small proportion of the total, and the original level can be restored by passing the current through a step-up transformer.

Distribution

As explained in the section on static transformers, distribution is by means of one live wire and one neutral wire (connected to earth). This method of distribution is much cheaper than if two live wires were used, as only one of the cables needs to be insulated, but the current is not earth-free. The cables may be carried across country by pylons or, in towns, taken underground enclosed in thick layers of insulation.

The Grid System

This is a system by which the electricity supplies throughout the greater part of the country are linked together. The supply is A.C. at 240 volts and a frequency of 50 cycles per second. A three-phase current is used. Each dynamo has three coils of wire which follow each other through the magnetic field so that a separate current is generated in each coil. One end of each coil is connected to a live distribution line while the other ends are connected together and to earth. Distribution of current is by three live cables, one from each of the dynamo coils, and one neutral cable, which is common to the three live wires. The current from the power stations is fed into a system of high tension cables extending through the country. Where a district is to be supplied the cables are tapped and the voltage stepped down at a transformer station. One end of each of the secondary coils of the transformer is connected to earth, and distribution throughout the area is again by three live wires and one neutral wire. Each consumer receives one of the live wires and the neutral wire. If it is a three-phase connection, consumer will receive three live wires and a neutral wire. As the current is alternating, the live wire is alternately negative and positive, the neutral wire being at zero potential throughout.

The grid system has the advantages that all areas supplied receive the same voltage and type of current; large demands in one area do not put an excessive load on any particular power station, and breakdown of one power station does not cut-off the supply to any area. It is not necessary for all the generators to be in operation all the time, so maintenance work is facilitated and the amount of stand-by equipment can be reduced.

22

Wiring of Houses

Distribution in a House

The current generated in the power station is supplied to the consumer by one live wire and one neutral wire, so the current is not earth-free. The current, on entering the house, passes through the main fuses and the meter. These are fixed by supply authority and should not be tampered with by the occupier. After this a main switch can be employed to cut-off the current supply to the house and the house main fuse is fixed which will blow if there is a short circuit or overload. Then a distribution box is fixed. In this box, the various circuits which are taken in parallel to each other are taken with separate MCB is attached for each circuit (Fig. 23.1). An ELCB is also fixed in this distribution box. This method of wiring is adopted so that each circuit receives the full voltage of the supply, the current in each is unaffected by that in the others, and they can be used independently of each other. Switches and fuses are wired in series with the supply points.

Light and Power Circuits

The circuits in the house can be divided into two categories, the light and the power circuits. The light circuits have a 5-ampere fuses for each four to six light points, and the wiring is designed to carry a slightly greater current than the fuses. The power circuits may be arranged similarly to the light circuits but with stronger wiring and with a fuse for each supply point. Thirteen-ampere fuses are used in modern wiring, 15-ampere fuses in systems of older construction, and the cables can carry a slightly greater current than the fuses. In addition to the above sub-circuits separate fuses may be used for different installations, such as, an electric cooker or immersion heater or, in a physiotherapy department, for certain equipment, such as, apparatus which uses a particularly large current.

The level of the current that flows in each circuit is determined by the apparatus, i.e., connected to it, being dependent on the EMF and the resistance of the circuit. The EMF is always constant as it is always determined by the source of supply. Therefore, the magnitude of the current depends on the resistance of the circuit: current varies inversely with resistance. All apparatus is marked with the voltage of the supply for which it is designed and the power (wattage) that it uses on that supply. Wattage is calculated by multiplying EMF by current, so if the wattage and EMF are known the magnitude of the current and the resistance of the apparatus can be calculated.

Switches

An electrical switch is any device used to interrupt the flow of electrons in a circuit. Switches are essentially binary devices: they are either completely on ('closed') or completely off ('open').

Types of Switches

- *Hand* switches are actuated by human touch.
- *Limit* switches are actuated by machine motion.
- *Process* switches are actuated by changes in some physical process (temperature, level, flow, etc.).

Hand switches are manufactured in several varieties.

Toggle switches (Fig. 22.1) are actuated by a lever angled in one of two or more positions. The common light switch used in household wiring is an example of a toggle switch. Even in physiotherapy department these switches are used. Most toggle switches will come to rest in any of their lever positions, while others have an internal spring mechanism returning the lever to a certain *normal* position, allowing for what is called 'momentary' operation.

When the switch is on, two metal blades fit into metal sockets. The principle is that when the switch is on the blades are gripped in the sockets and the circuit is completed. When the circuit is broken, a spring ensures the sudden separation of the sockets and blades, if they were parted slowly, arcing might occur, and the intense heat would gradually burn away the metal contacts.

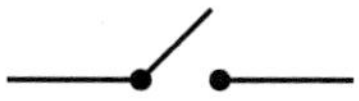

Fig. 22.1: Toggle switch

Pushbutton switches (Fig. 22.2) are two-position devices actuated with a button, i.e., pressed and released. Most pushbutton switches have an internal spring mechanism returning the button to its 'out', or 'unpressed', position, for momentary operation.

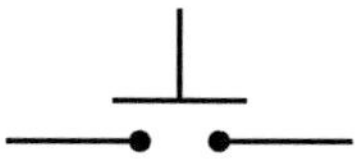

Fig. 22.2: Pushbutton switch

Selector switches (Fig. 22.3) are actuated with a rotary knob or lever of some sort to select one of two or more positions. Like the toggle switch, selector switches can either rest in any of their positions or contain spring-return mechanisms for momentary operation.

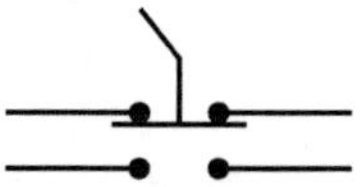

Fig. 22.3: Selector switch

A joystick switch (Fig 22.4) is actuated by a lever free to move in more than one axis of motion. One or more of several switch contact mechanisms are actuated depending on which way the lever is pushed, and sometimes by how far it is pushed. The circle-and-dot notation on the switch symbol represents the direction of joystick lever motion required to actuate the contact. Joystick hand switches are commonly used for crane and robot control.

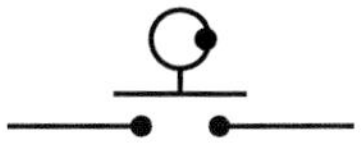

Fig. 22.4: Joystick switch

Description of limit and process switches are beyond the scope of this text book.

There is a switch for each light and power point and it is most satisfactory if this breaks both wires of the circuit. When this is not so, the switch should interrupt the live wire, otherwise connection to the live wire can be made even when the switch is turned off, and the danger of earth shock exists.

Plug and Sockets

AC power plugs and sockets are devices that allow electrically operated equipment to be connected to the primary alternating current (AC) power supply in a building. Generally, the plug is the movable connector attached to an electrically operated device's mains cable, and the socket is fixed on equipment or a building structure and connected to an energised electrical circuit. The plug has protruding pins or prongs or, in US terminology, blades (referred to as male) that fit into matching slots or holes (called female) in the sockets. There are currently 15 types of electrical outlet plugs in use today, each of which has been assigned a letter by the US Department of Commerce International Trade Administration (ITA), starting with A and moving through the alphabet till the letter 0. Type C (Fig. 22.5) and D (Fig. 22.6) is commonly used in India. The advantage is that it has a physical interface so that one can switch it on and off with a switch.

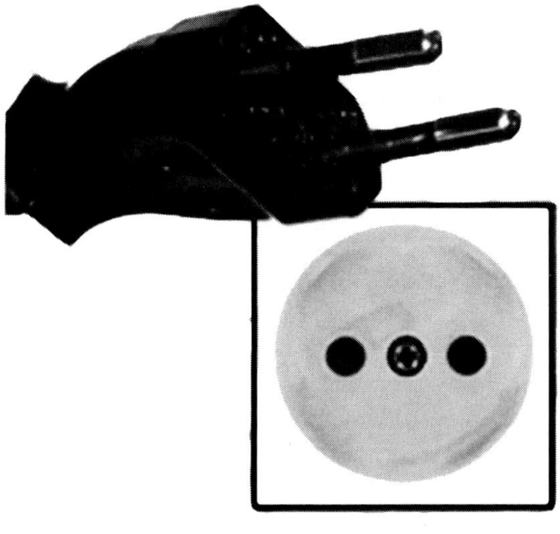

Fig. 22.5: Type C

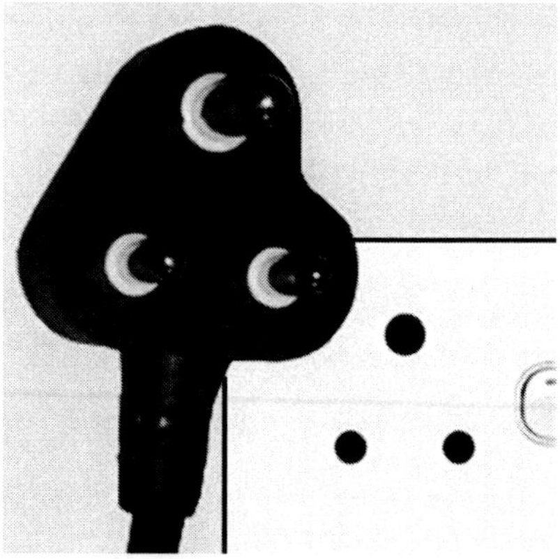

Fig. 22.6: Type D

The Electrotherapy apparatus working on a power circuit should be connected to the supply by a three-pin wall-plug (Type D). The pins to fit into power sockets are arranged in a triangle, two being similar and the third (the earth pin) either larger or differently spaced from the others, so that the plug can be inserted into the socket in one way only. The two similar pins are for connection of the apparatus circuit to the supply, and are marked 'L' and 'N' for the live and neutral wires. Some plugs incorporate a fuse on the live wire. This must not be capable of carrying more than the 13 amperes that the main wiring is designed to carry but should be selected according to the current used by the apparatus which it connects to the supply: in this way, it safeguards both the main wiring and the apparatus circuit. Normally, the brown wire is connected to the pin marked 'L', the blue wire to that marked 'N' and the green-and-yellow wire to the third pin, which marked 'E'. The wire connected to the pin marked 'E' is for connection of the apparatus casing to earth. The socket into which it fits is earthed and the other end of the wire is connected to the apparatus casing. The third pin may operate a switch which disconnects the other two sockets from the source of supply when the plug is withdrawn, or a shutter which prevents contact with these sockets.

23

Safety Devices

INTRODUCTION

Safety devices are Three Prong plugs, Fuses, MCB, Earth-leakage circuit breaker, Residual current circuit breaker and Grounding. Surge Protector is also considered as safety device which is designed to protect electrical devices from voltage spikes (e.g., a lightning strike). It attempts to block the voltage supplied to a device above a safe threshold (Fig. 23.1).

Three Prong Plugs

Apparatus working on a power circuit should be connected to the supply by a three-pin wall plug. This three-pin plug consists of live, neutral and the earth pin. Details are covered in preceding chapter.

Fuses

A fuse is an electrical safety device that has the capability to protect a circuit from excessive current. It is designed to allow current through the circuit, but in the event that the current exceeds some maximum value it will open, severing the circuit.

Definition: Fuse is a safety device used to protect the circuit and minimise damage to the lowest possible level.

Principle: A relatively short piece of conducting material, with a cross-sectional area insufficient to carry currents quite as high as those which may be permitted to flow in the protected circuit, is sacrificed when necessary, to prevent healthy parts of the circuit being damaged and to limit the damage to faulty sections or items to the lowest possible level.

Classification

1. *High voltage fuse*: Commonly used to protect transformers.
2. *Low voltage fuse* (also called as automotive fuses), for vehicles also called as blade fuses.

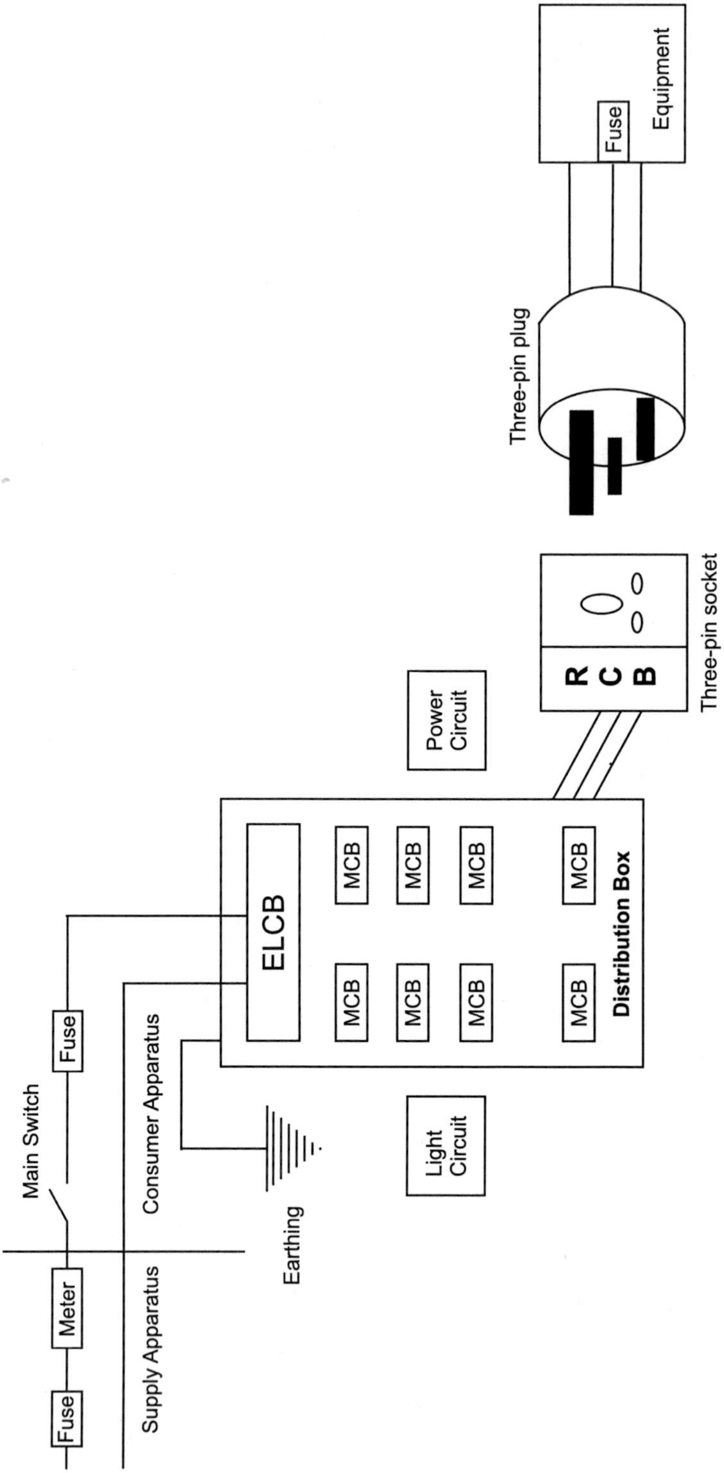

Fig. 23.1: Overview of safety devices

3. *Cartridge fuse or Enclosed fuse or Miniature fuse*, are used in Physiotherapy department (Fig. 23.2).
4. *Porcelain fuse* used as main fuse in houses and hospitals (Fig. 23.3).
5. *Resettable fuse* can be used for many number of times.
6. *Thermal fuse* used in coffee maker or hair dryer.

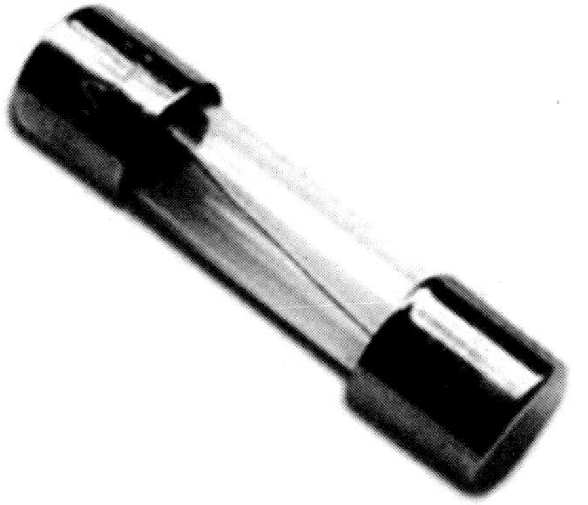

Fig. 23.2: Cartridge fuse

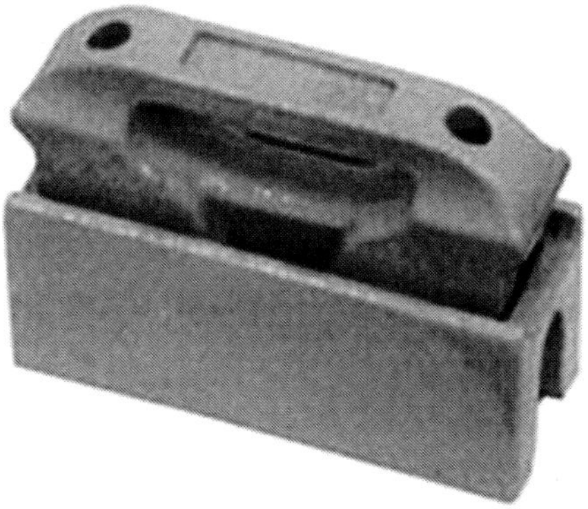

Fig. 23.3: Porcelain fuse

Construction and Working

- Fuse consists of a metal strip or wire fuse element, of small cross-section compared to the circuit conductors, mounted between a pair of electrical terminals, and (usually) enclosed by a non-combustible housing.
- The fuse element is made of zinc, copper, silver, aluminum.
- The fuse is arranged in series to carry all the current passing through the protected circuit. The resistance of the element generates heat due to the current flow.
- If too high a current flows, the element rises to a higher temperature and either directly melts, or else melts a soldered joint within the fuse, opening the circuit.

- If a fuse blows, the apparatus which caused the damage should be disconnected and the main supply switched off.

  Functions: Used for over current protection.

  Causes for it:

- Short-circuit
- Overloading
- Mismatch loads
- Device failures.

The blowing of a fuse is the result of the passage of too great a current. This may arise in various ways:

- The current will exceed the permitted level if the apparatus connected is of too low a resistance, i.e., too high a wattage, such as, a 2000 Watt electric device on a light circuit.
- If several parallel circuits are taken from one supply point, the total current obtained is the sum of that in the individual circuits and may blow the fuse: this is liable to occur when adaptors are used to take extra circuits from a light or power point.
- A short-circuit in the wiring or apparatus causes a reduction of the resistance and a large current passes. Such a short-circuit may occur if the insulation round the flex connecting the apparatus to the source of supply becomes worn, so that the two supply wires come in contact with each other, or as a result of a connection between the live wire and earth.

Advantages

- Cheap
- Zero maintenance
- Simplicity in operation
- Ability to interrupt short-circuit without making noise or smoke.

Disadvantages

- During short-circuit or overload once fuse blows off replacing of fuse takes time. During this period, the circuit will loose power.
- When fuses are connected in series, it is difficult to discriminate the fuse unless the fuse has significant difference.

Application in Physiotherapy

The most common type of fuse used in physiotherapy department is the cartridge in which the fusible element is made of silver wire and runs between metal caps through a tube of glass or other suitable non-inflammable insulating material. It is held in position by metal contact clips. The whole tube is replaced when necessary. In a physiotherapy department, fuses should be included in the circuit of each piece of apparatus used for the treatment of patients, in addition to those in the department wiring. If a fault occurs, blowing of the apparatus fuse affects only one patient, whereas if one of the department fuses blows, the current is cut-off from all patients receiving treatment from this section of the wiring.

MCB AND MCCB

MCB (Miniature Circuit Breaker): It is used for up to 100 Amps in the motor feeders.

MCCB (Moulded Case Circuit Breaker): It is used for 250–800 Amps in the motor feeders. Only MCBs will be discussed here.

Definition

Circuit breakers are devices that protect circuits from overload current conditions. They do the same job as fuses, but they are not destroyed when activated. They are more expensive to put in than fuses, but since components rarely need to be replaced may be cheaper in the long-term. Circuit breakers are often considered safer since the user can't as easily disable them (like putting the wrong size fuse in place).

Function

They are designed to protect the wiring in a building. It detects a fault in the wiring and interrupts the flow of current. A circuit breaker may 'trip' when an electrical receptacle has become overloaded. One can reset the circuit breaker to restore current flow. (Note: Make sure that the circuit is no longer overloaded before resetting the circuit breaker). If the circuit will not reset by turning all the way off and back on, then better to contact an electrician.

Table 23.1: Fuse versus MCB comparison

	Fuse	***MCB***
Advantages	Less cost Simpler *Less convenient:* The blown fuse must be replaced with a new device.	It automatically switches off the electrical circuit during abnormal condition (over load and faulty condition). As the switch operating knob comes at its off position during tripping, the faulty zone of the electrical circuit can easily be identified. But in case of fuse, fuse wire should be checked by opening fuse grip or cut-out from fuse base, for confirming the blow of fuse wire. MCB is much more sensitive to over current than fuse. MCB is quick work against short-circuit, earth leakage, overloading and under voltage. MCB is reliable.
Disadvantages	Replacing a fuse without isolating the circuit first (most building wiring designs do not provide individual isolation switches for each fuse) can be dangerous in itself, particularly if the fault is a short-circuit.	The cost of MCB is greater than fuse. The cost of on MCB distribution board is greater than rewireable fuse board.

EARTH-LEAKAGE CIRCUIT BREAKER (ELCB)

Introduction

An earth-leakage circuit breaker (ELCB) is a safety device used in electrical installations with high earth impedance to prevent shock. It detects small stray voltages on the metal enclosures of electrical equipment, and interrupts the circuit if a dangerous voltage is detected.

Construction and Working

These devices sense a voltage to decide the earth leakage. A single-phase voltage ELCB will have six terminals. Line in and out, neutral in and out, earth (E), and fault (F). Metal body of the load is connected to the fault terminal of ELCB and earth terminal is connected to the ground. For normal working, voltage across the trip coil is zero, because, the body of the load is isolated from the supply line. When an earth fault occurs on the load, due to the contact of line wire to the metal body, a current will flow through F to the ground. This current will set up a voltage across the trip coil, which is connected between E and F. The energized trip coil will trip the circuit to protect the load device and the user. ELCB detects a rise in potential between the protected interconnected metalwork (equipment frames, conduits, enclosures) and a distant isolated earth reference electrode.

Function

The main purpose of earth leakage protectors is to prevent injury to humans and animals due to electric shock.

Advantages

They are less sensitive to fault conditions.

Disadvantages

Disadvantages includes:

- Wire break in the fault to load section or earth to ground section will results, a failure in operation of ELCB, and user may get severe electric shock, during earth fault.
- Requirement of an additional third wire from the load to the ELCB.
- Separate devices cannot be grounded individually.
- The voltage-operated ELCB are the requirement for a second connection, and the possibility that any additional connection to earth on the protected system can disable the detector.

RESIDUAL CURRENT CIRCUIT BREAKER (RCCB OR RCD OR RCBO OR GFCI OR ALCI)

Introduction

A residual-current device (RCD), or residual-current circuit breaker (RCCB), is a device to quickly disconnect current to prevent serious harm from an ongoing electric shock. In the United States and Canada, the device is more commonly known as a ground fault circuit interrupter (GFCI), ground fault interrupter (GFI) or an appliance leakage current interrupter (ALCI). In the United Kingdom, these are better known by their initials RCD, and a combined RCD + MCB are known as a RCBO (residual-current circuit breaker with overcurrent protection).

Principle

Residual current breaker (RCB) works on the assumption that the current going to the electronics device must come out from the neutral wire, if there is no other way for current flow. In simple words, RCB measures the current going inside the connected device and coming out from the device. If both of these current are equal, then there would no problem with the normal functionality of the device. This device is also known as Current Operated ELCB.

Construction and Working

RCCB consists of a three-winding transformer, which has two primary windings and one secondary winding. Neutral and line wires act as the two primary windings. A wire wound coil is the secondary winding. The current through the secondary winding is zero at the balanced condition. In balance condition, the flux due to the current through the phase wire will be neutralized by the current through the neutral wire, since the current, which flows from the phase will be returned back to the neutral. When a fault occurs, a small current will flow to the ground also. This makes an unbalance between line and neutral current and that creates an unbalanced magnetic field. This induces a current through the secondary winding, which is connected to the sensing circuit. This will sense the leakage and send signal to tripping system.

Types

RCDs can be fixed, socket outlet and portable.

Fixed RCDs: These are installed in the consumer unit (fuse box) and can provide protection to individual or groups of circuits. A fixed RCD provides the highest level of protection as it protects all the wiring and the sockets on a circuit, and any connected appliances.

Socket-Outlet RCDs: These are special socket-outlets with an RCD built into them which can be used in place of a standard socket-outlet. This type of RCD provides protection only to the person in contact with equipment, including its lead, plugged into the special socket-outlet.

Portable RCDs: These plugs into any standard socket-outlet. An appliance can then be plugged into the RCD. They are useful when neither fixed nor socket-outlet RCDs are available but, as with socket-outlet RCDs, they provide protection only to the person in contact with the equipment, including its lead, plugged into the portable RCD.

Uses

A ground fault circuit interrupt is a device designed to detect a tiny mismatch in currents (going into and out of the circuit), in order to prevent electrocution. They are mandatory in bathrooms and kitchens, and anywhere else in a house where water may come in contact with an electric circuit. RCDs offer a level of personal protection that ordinary fuses and circuit-breakers cannot provide. An RCD constantly monitors the electric current flowing through one or more circuits, it is used to protect. If it detects electricity flowing down an unintended path, such as, through a person who has touched a live part, the RCD will switch the circuit off very quickly, significantly reducing the risk of death or serious injury.

Advantages

1. If there is no connection between the ground and the enclosure of the device, and a person touches the metallic body of that device. In this case, incoming and outgoing current will be different and RCB will Trip in contrast with ELCB.
2. Functionality of RCB (Residual Current Breaker) does not effect by lightning strikes.
3. It does not trip falsely.

Disadvantages

1. An RCD does not provide protection against unexpected or dangerously high current when current is flowing in the usual wires in the circuit, therefore, it cannot replace a fuse or protect against overheating or fire risk due to overcurrent (overload) or short circuits if the fault does not lead to current leakage. Therefore, RCDs are often used or integrated as a single product along with some kind of circuit breaker, such as, a fuse or miniature circuit breaker (MCB).
2. RCDs also cannot detect the situation where a human accidentally touches both conductors at the same time, since the flow of current through an expected device, an unexpected route, or a human, are indistinguishable if the current returns through the expected conductor.

GROUNDING (Fig. 23.4)

There are two kinds of grounding:

1. **Electrical circuit or system grounding:** One conductor of the circuit is intentionally grounded to earth. It protects circuit from lightning, or other high voltage contact.
2. **Electrical equipment grounding:** All metal frames and enclosures of equipment are grounded by a permanent connection. The equipment grounding conductor provides a path for dangerous fault current to return to the system ground at the supply source should a fault occur.

   The earthing of the apparatus casing is a precaution against earth shock. If the insulation of the live wire is worn out, this comes in contact with metal casing. If this connection is through a person he may receive a shock. However, if apparatus is earthed, the current passes through this low resistance circuit (between the casing and earth). Since this current flow is great, the fuse on the live wire will blow. This stops the current flow and gives warning of the defect. Such a circuit is the point at which the insulation is worn being indicated by the arrow. Exceptions to the need to earth apparatus-casing occur when the casing is of non-conducting material and when the apparatus is 'double insulated', making a connection between the live wire and the casing virtually impossible.

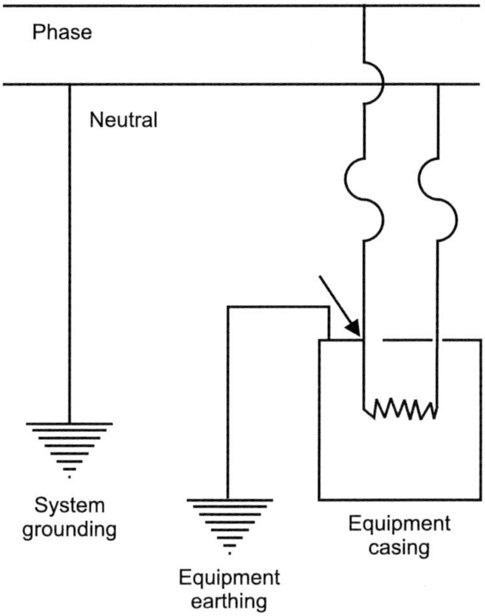

Fig. 23.4: System grounding and equipment grounding

24

Electric Shock

DEFINITION

A shock is a painful stimulation of sensory nerves caused by sudden flow, cessation or variation in the current passing through the body.

Factors affecting the severity of the shock:

1. Ohm's law: Higher EMF and lower resistance results in more shock.
   - V/I = R, V/R = I.
   - ↑V/↓R = I↑ (Voltage is directly proportional to current and resistance is inversely proportional to Current).
2. Wet hand than dry hand.
3. Path taken by the current.
4. AC compared to DC.
   Prolonged tetanic contraction makes it impossible for the victim to let go out of the current.

Physiological Effects

- Up to 20–40 mA, labored breathing.
- Up to 100 mA muscular paralysis, ventricular fibrillation, cannot let go condition.
- 100–200 mA, unconsciousness, cardiac and respiratory arrest.
- Above 200 mA death.

Types of Shock

- Macro shock
- Micro shock
- Earth shock
- Major shock

- Minor shock.

Macro Shock: If the current flow is from body surface through the skin into the body, a large amount of current is needed to produce a shock.

Micro Shock: If the current bypasses the surface of the body and enters the heart through myocardial electrode or transverse catheter or through the pacemaker. In this case, a minute current can produce fatal shock without the patient experiencing any sensation.

Earth Shock: When a shock is due to the connection between live wire of main and earth.

Minor Shock: Results in skin changes.

Major Shock: Results in unconsciousness.

Causes of Shock

- Touching the metal case: Short-circuit in the casing due to moisture, dust and deterioration.
- Leakage: Lack of insulation around the live wire.
- Two pin connection: Lack of ground connection.
- Badly serviced medical apparatus.

Clinical Features

Clinical Features of Minor Shock

- First 12 hours skin will become white surrounding by hyperemia (reddening) followed by edema. and inflammation followed by widening of demarked area.
- Whitish skin changes into black due to necrosis.
- Followed by death of fat, muscles and tendon.

Clinical Features of Major Shock

- Signs of cardiac arrest: Absence of pulse, Unconsciousness.
- Sign of respiratory arrest: Absence of chest wall movement.
- Changes in tissue.
- Coagulation necrosis.
- Damage to tunica media.
- Thrombosis.

If severity is more it may lead to death (Fig. 24.1).

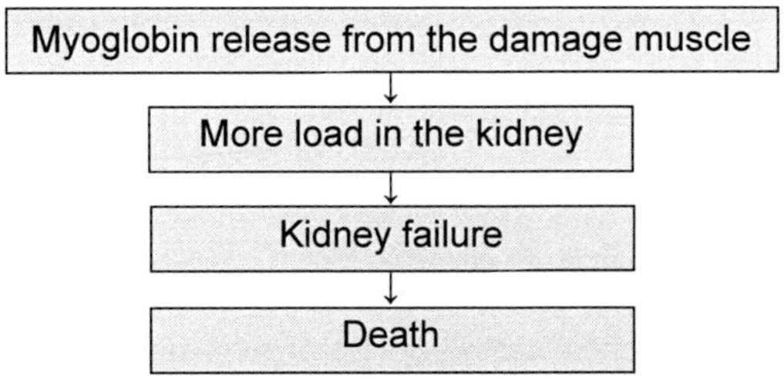

Fig. 24.1: Cause of death due to shock

Precaution

Equipments Used

- Use of three-pin plug instead of two-pin.
- Insulation around the conductor.
- Use of MCB/RCB/ELCB.
- Don't use same power outlet for two machines.
- Avoid the use of extension box.
- Use of fuse.
- Proper earthing or ground connection.
- Never pull the plug out of the socket by pulling the wire.
- Unplug the equipment at the end of day's off.
- After Rx, intensity should be reduced.
- Check power.
- Regular service.

Positioning of Equipment

- The equipment should be placed on wooden surfaces.
- All couches should be of wood/plastic.
- IFT machine should be 4 m far from SWD and MWD.
- Antennae of the MWD should be directed to the wall.
- Equipments should be 10 m far from ECG and pacemaker.
- Don't place electrical equipment next to the water.

Patient's Precautions

- Check for contraindications.
- Testing of machine.
- Check for patient's sensation.
- Warm the patients about the danger.
- Install the warming boards.

Therapist Precautions

- Wearing the foot wear.
- Always off the switch and unplug the socket after treatment.

Treatment of Shock Victims

- Disconnect the victim from the source of supply by wooden piece.
- Equipment should be switched off.
- Contact with the patient with a layer of insulating material.

- Reassurance to the victim.
- Rest should be given.
- Give water to prevent dehydration.
- Avoid hot drinks (otherwise lead to tachycardia) (Fig. 24.2).
- Refer to the physician.

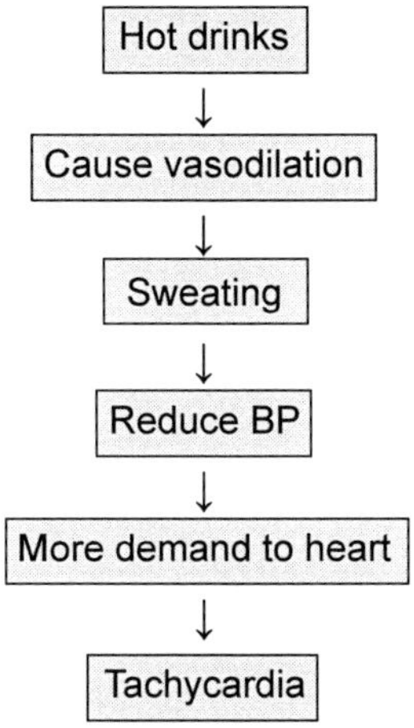

Fig. 24.2: Sequence of events with administration of hot drinks

Management of Unconscious Patient

- If patient is unconscious, there is no sign of cardiac and respiratory arrest then put the patient in rescue positions, i.e., side lying.
- Loosen all the tight clothing for respiration.
- If patient in unconscious and there is sign of cardiac and respiratory arrest then perform CPR (cardiopulmonary resuscitation). Basic steps administered are ABCD, i.e., Airway, Breathing, Circulation and Defibrillation.
- Oxygen therapy.
- Refer to the physician.

25

Electrical Burns and Chemical Burns

Burns are injuries to tissues caused by heat, friction, electricity, radiation, or chemicals. Two types of burns can occur with the application of electrotherapy currents. They are chemical burn and electrical burn.

CHEMICAL BURN

Chemical burn is produced by the application of DC. Destruction of tissue takes place, the burn appears as grey spot surrounded by reddened area. There is coagulation of tissue at anode and liquefaction at cathode. Acid formation under anode and alkaline formation under cathode. A long duration pulses produce more burn compared to short duration pulses. A uniphasic pulse produces more burn compared to biphasic pulse. The order of producing the severity of burns is as follows:

Sinusoidal currents < SDIDC (Faradic) < LDIDC (Galvanic) < TDC or current used for iontophoresis

Treatment of Chemical Burn

- Healing takes place by secondary intention.
- Area should be kept dry.
- It should not become infected so it is protected by dry sterile gauze.
- The healing is accelerated by infrared therapy.

Prevention of Chemical Burn

- Use of a reversing switch after the treatment in order to change the direction of current.
- Change the polarity of electrode after the treatment.
- Increase the intensity gradually.
- Check the sensation.
- Lint pad should be 16 layered.

- Reduce current density by using large electrode.
- Avoid direct contact of metal electrode with skin.
- Use the coupling media so that electrochemical changes takes place outside the tissue.

Electrical Burn

Electrical burn happens due to the following causes:

- Due to a shock.
- When the body becomes contact with a metal electrode directly.
- From the junction of lead wire with rubber electrode when it is loose.
- If point of contact of pen electrode is too much pressed.
- Through the open wounds.
- Through scar marks.

Prevention and management is given in the Chapter 24.

26

Types of Currents and Its Effects on Body

TYPES OF CURRENTS

Therapeutic currents can be classified on the basis of direction, frequency, voltage, amperage and based on effects. A simple classification of low frequency currents is detailed in Figure 26.1.

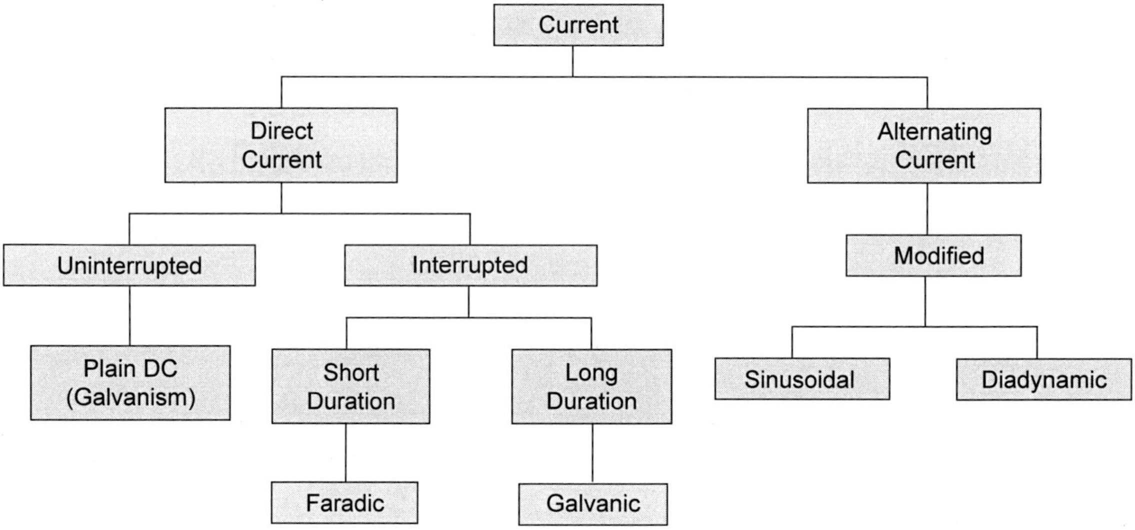

Fig. 26.1: Classification of low frequency currents

A. Classification Based on Frequency

1. **Low frequency current:** 10–1000 Hertz
   (a) Modified AC
      (i) Sinusoidal current
      (ii) Diadynamic current

   (b) Galvanic current
   (c) Faradic current
   (d) TENS
2. **Medium frequency current:** 1000–10000 Hz
   (a) Russian current
   (b) Rebox current
   (c) Interferential current
3. **High frequency current:** Above 10000 Hz
   (a) MWD (Micro wave diathermy)
   (b) SWD (Sort wave diathermy)
   (c) LWD (Long wave diathermy)
   (d) Ultrasound

B. Classification Based on Electrophysiological Effects
(Described later in this chapter)

1. Electrochemical effects.
2. Electrothermal effects.
3. Electrophysical effects.

C. Classification Based on the Directional and Waveforms

1. **Direct Current (DC):** This is continuous unidirectional flow of charged particles with duration of at least 1 second. One electrode is always the anode (+) and one is always the cathode (-) for the entire event. There is a build-up of charge since it is moving in one direction causing a strong chemical effect on the tissue under the electrode.
2. **Alternating Current (AC):** This is uninterrupted bidirectional flow of charged particles and changing direction at least once per second. Electrodes continuously changes polarity each cycle, therefore, no build-up of charge under the electrodes. Often used in interferential or Russian commercial stimulators.
3. **Pulsed Current (Pulsed):** This can be unidirectional (like DC) or bidirectional (like AC). Flow of charged particles stops periodically for less than 1 second before the next event. Pulses can occur individually or in a series.

D. Classification Based on Strength of Currents

1. **Micro Currents:** Current lesser than 1 mA.
2. **Macro Currents:** Currents greater than 1 mA.

Physiologic Responses to Electrical Current

The normal physiological response to electrical current may be excitatory or non-excitatory. This series of changes may happen from cellular level to tissue level to segmental level and can go up to systemic level. The effects of electrical current passing through the various tissues of the body may be:

- Electrothermal.
- Electrochemical.
- Electrophysiological.

Electrothermal Effect: All electrical currents cause a rise in temperature in a conducting tissue. The tissues of the body possess varying degrees of resistance, and those of higher resistance should heat up more when electrical current passes through. As indicated, the diathermies generate a continuous high-frequency electrical current that is designed to produce a tissue temperature increase. The electrical currents used for stimulation of nerve and muscle have a relatively low average current flow that produces minimal thermal effects.

Electrophysiological Effect: Basically, electrical currents are used to produce either muscle contractions or modification of pain impulses through effects on the motor and sensory nerves. This function is dependent to a great extent on selecting the appropriate treatment parameters based on the principles identified in this chapter.

Electrochemical Effect: Electrical currents are also used to produce chemical effects. Most biologic tissue contains negatively and positively charged ions. A direct current flow will cause migration of these charged particles toward the pole of opposite polarity. At the positive pole the negatively charged particles cause an acid reaction in which there is coagulation of protein and hardening of the tissues. At the negative pole the positively charged particles produce an alkaline reaction, liquefying protein, and causing softening of the tissues.

27

Nerve Muscle Physiology

RESTING MEMBRANE POTENTIAL

Definition

It is the potential difference across the membrane at rest. It is also termed as trans-membrane potential or polarized rate of the membrane. In the polarized state inside the cell is more negative while outside the cell is more positive. It is because of unequal distribution of ions across the membrane. In extracellular fluid (ECF), there is increased concentration of Na^+ and Cl^- ions while in intracellular fluid (ICF), there is increased concentration of K^+ and protein$^-$ ions. This difference in the composition between the ICF and the ECF produces a potential difference across the membrane.

Two conditions are necessary for the membrane potential to develop:

(1) The membrane must be semi-permeable, allowing ions of one charge to diffuse through pores more readily than ions of the opposite charge; and

(2) The concentration of the diffusible ions must be greater on one side of the membrane than on the other side.

Mechanism that Maintain the Unequal Distribution of Ions

- The activity of K^+ leak channels at rest. At rest a number of potassium leak channels are open causing K^+ ion to move into the ICF. Thereby maintaining the negativity or polarized state of the cell.
- The activity of the Na^+/K^+ pump: It pumps out three sodium ions and pumps in two potassium ions.

ACTION POTENTIAL

Introduction

Action potential occurs only in the excitable tissue. The transmembrane potential is present in all the cells of the body whereas action potential is present only in the excitable tissue of the body, i.e., Nerve cell and Muscle cell.

Definition

It is brief change in potential towards positivity followed by a change towards negativity.

It involves two processes:

- Change in membrane potential towards positivity, this is called *depolarization.*
- Change in membrane potential towards negativity, this is called *repolarization.*

IONIC BASIS OF ACTION POTENTIAL

Action potential has four phases. Following are the phases:

1. Phase Zero/Local Current

- Value: –70 mV to –55 mV
- Cause is detailed in Figure 27.1

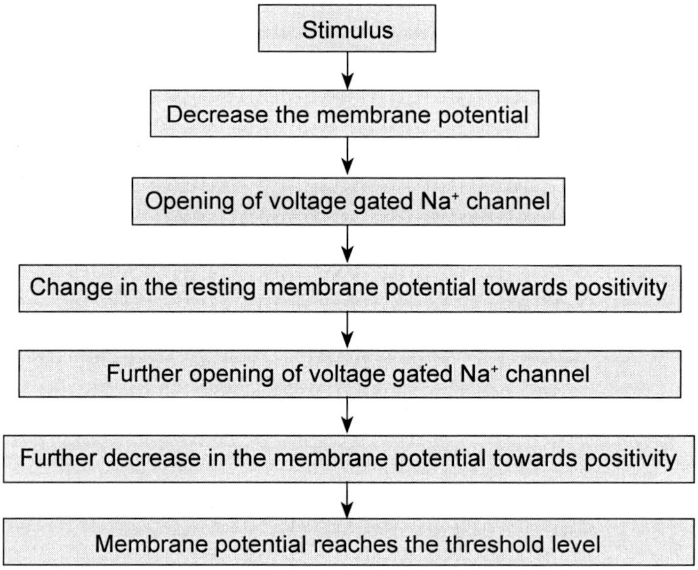

Fig. 27.1: Events take place at Phase zero

2. Phase 1

It refers to the phase where there is rapid decrease in the membrane potential towards positivity. This produces spike potential.

- Value: –55 mV to + 30 mV
- Cause is detailed in Figure 27.2

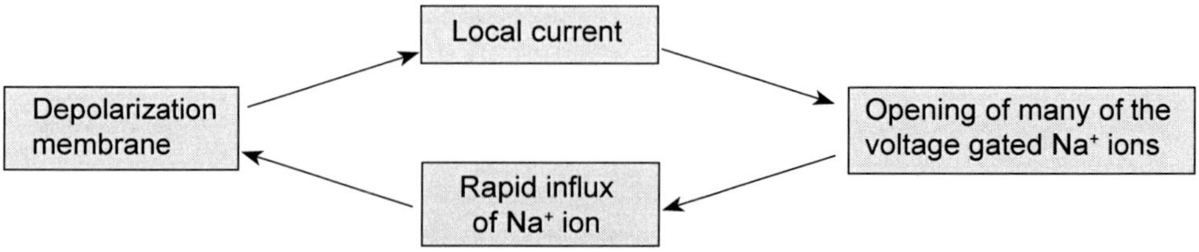

Fig 27.2: Events that takes place in Phase 1

3. Phase 2

Definition

It is a phase in the action potential where there is the change in the membrane potential back to negativity.

Value: +30 mV to –70 mV

Cause

(i) Inactivation of voltage gated Na channel

(ii) Opening of voltage gated K^+ channel results in efflux of K^+ ion.

Cause no. (i) and (ii) result in the increase of negativity inside the cell thereby Repolarization.

4. Phase 3

Definition

It is a phase where the membrane potential becomes more negative than its resting membrane potential.

Value: –70mV to –80/–90 mV.

Cause

(i) Voltage gated sodium channel are closed which results in absence in the influx of Na^+ ions.

(ii) Voltage gated K^+ channel continues to remain open which results in efflux of K^+ ions continues even after reaching resting membrane potential.

This causes membrane potential to become more negative than the resting membrane potential.

A summary of formation of action potential is listed in Figure 27.3 and opening and closing of gated channels are listed in Figure 27.4.

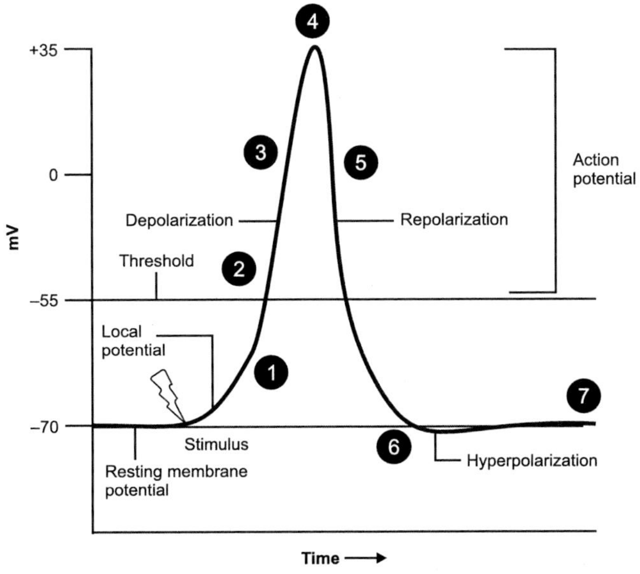

Fig. 27.3: Formation of action potential

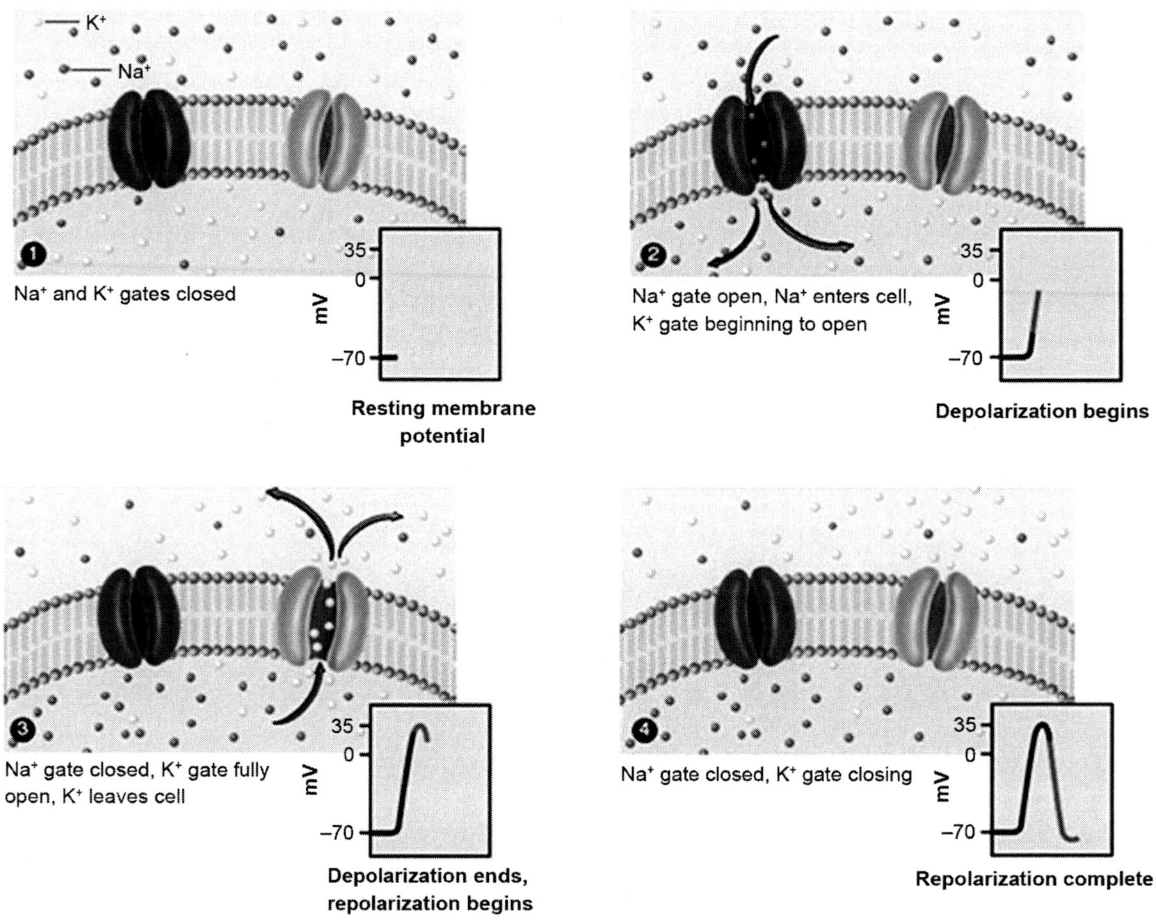

Fig. 27.4: Opening and closing gated channels during development of action potential

1. Development of local potential
2. Threshold of excitation
3. Depolarization
4. Peak action potential
5. Repolarization
6. Hyperpolarization
7. Return to rest.

Electrical Stimulation of Nerve

Electrically stimulating a nerve will have same sequence as that of a voluntary contraction. A summary of events is listed in Figure 27.5.

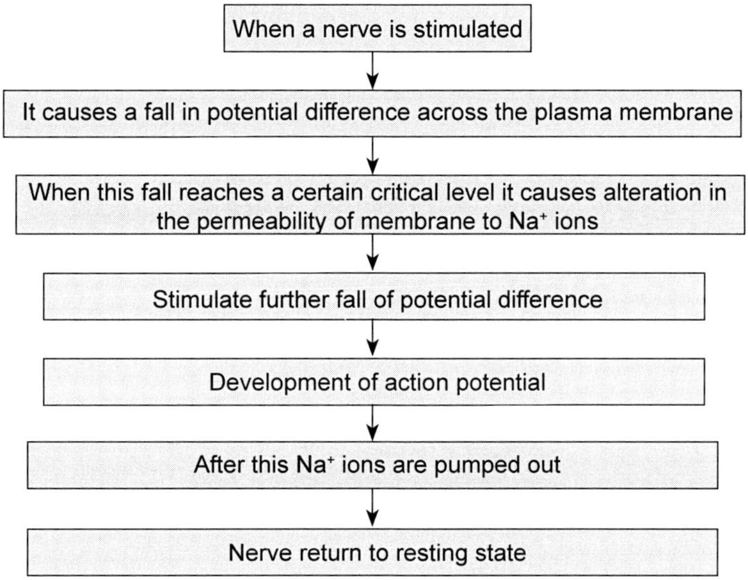

Fig. 27.5: Electrical stimulation of a nerve

Propagation of Action Potential

Action potential can be propagated along the length of the nerve either by local electron flow or by saltatory conduction. Their differences are listed in Table 27.1.

Table 27.1: Difference between local electron flow and saltatory conduction

Saltatory conduction	*Local electron flow*
Occurs in myelinated nerve fiber	Occurs in non-myelinated nerve fiber
Rapid conduction of impulse	Slow conduction of impulse
It is the intermittent conduction (node to node)	It is the continuous conduction
Conduction of impulses from one node of ranvier to other	Point to point conduction of the impulse/electric current through entire axon

Local electron flow: The difference of potential between active and the resting part of the nerve causes the local electron flow between the active and adjacent part of the nerve. These changes are propagated along the length of the nerve fiber (Fig. 27.6).

Saltatory conduction: The impulses jump from one node of ranvier another node of ranvier (Fig. 27.7).

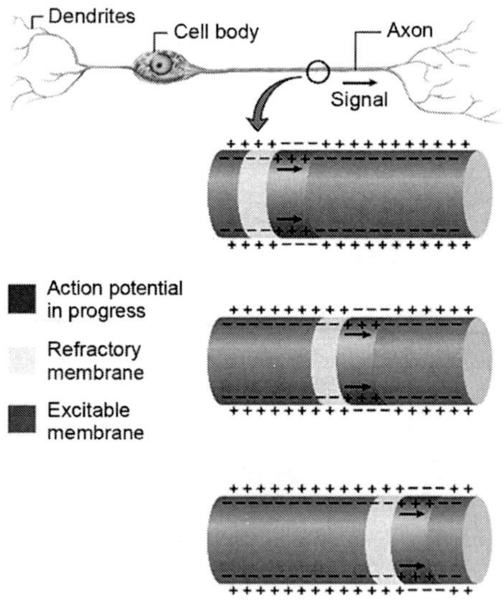

Fig. 27.6: Local electron flow

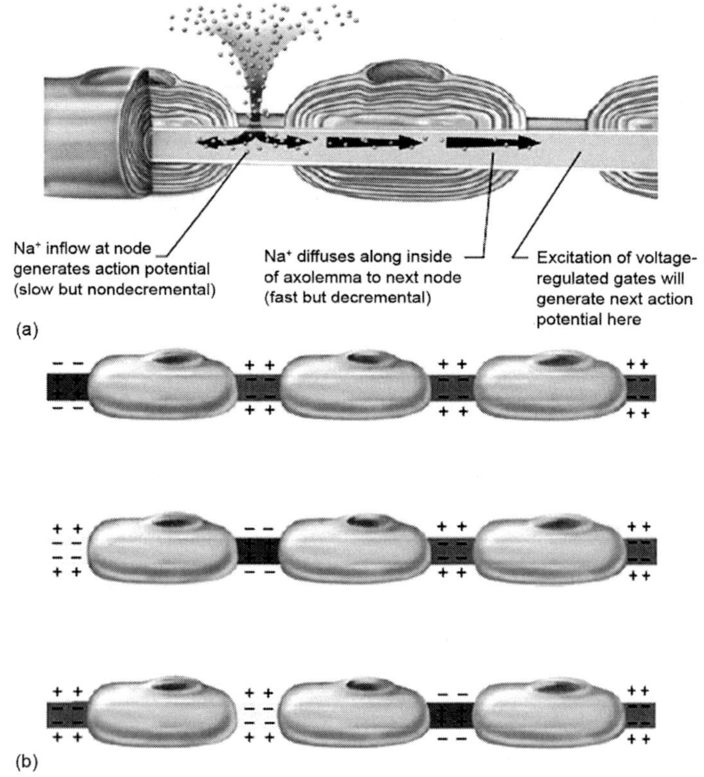

Fig. 27.7: Saltatory conduction

Accommodation or Adaptation

When a constant current flows, the nerve adapt itself to the current such that there is no initiation of impulse which is known as accommodation. The nerve has the property of accommodation whereas the muscle does not have the property of accommodation. Fast rising pulse will never produce accommodation so to stimulate a nerve a rectangular pulse is preferred. Slow rising pulse is preferred for stimulating a muscle since the muscle does not have property of accommodation. The current which rises or falls suddenly is more effective in initiating an impulse than it changes slowly. If accommodation takes place greater current is required for subsequent contraction.

Hot Spot

Q. Why a nerve is easily stimulated first followed by a muscle?

Ans.: The resting membrane is relatively not completely impermeable to sodium ions (Na) which is held in greater concentration outside the cells. In contrast, the resting membrane is significantly more permeable to potassium (K) which is held in greater concentration inside the cell. Due to concentration gradients small amount of sodium leak into the cell and potassium leaks out of the cell. ATP driven sodium potassium pump helps to maintain the separation of ions by transporting Na and 2K back into the cell. This results in negativity (due to less positive ions inside). The RMP of different tissues are as follows: Nerve = –70 mV, muscle = –90 mV, cardiac = –85 mV due to relative permeability to sodium and potassium. Since RMP of nerve is less negative compared to a muscle, a nerve is always stimulated first followed by muscle.

28

Basics of Application of Currents

Difference Between Voluntary Contraction and Electrically Evoked Muscle Contraction in Motor Unit Recruitment

Response of electrically evoked muscle contraction is different from voluntary contraction which is detailed in Table 28.1. Hanneman, *et al.* proposed size principle which states that the order of recruitment in a normal voluntary contraction is from small to large nerve fiber diameters. Slow fatigue resistant muscle fibers are innervated by smaller diameter nerve fibers whereas fast fatigue muscle fibers have larger diameter motor nerves controlling them. With electrical stimulation, the order is reversed. Fiber diameter is a key factor as depolarization depends on the potential difference between two adjacent nodes of ranvier and spacing between adjacent nodes is proportional to the fiber diameter. Also the distance of the nerve fiber from stimulating electrode and the nerve fiber diameter determines the order of recruitment.

Table 28.1: Difference between voluntary contraction and electrically stimulated muscle contraction

Voluntary contraction	***Electrically evoked***
Active	***Passive***
Temporal motor unit recruitment Asynchronous firing	Temporal motor unit recruitment Synchronous firing
Type I fibers (slow fibers) are recruited more as compared to type II fibers	Type II fibers (fast fibers) are recruited more compared to type I fibers
Fatigue is less	Fatigue is more
Spatial motor unit recruitment is small to large	Spatial motor unit recruitment is large to small
Force of contraction is graded	Force of contraction is not graded
Force of contraction is increased partly by increasing the firing rate of the activated motor unit and partly by recruiting more motor unit	Force of contraction is increased by increasing the intensity
Action potential moved away from the nerve cell body	Action potential generated in two directions, away from the cell body and back toward the cell body

Difference Between Innervated Muscle and Denervated Muscle

Difference is detailed in Table 28.2.

Table 28.2: Difference between innervated muscle and denervated muscle

Innervated muscle	*Denervated muscle*
Muscle with an intact nerve is innervated muscle.	A muscle with a detached nerve is called denervated muscle.
Faradic current is used for innervated muscle.	Galvanic current is used for denervated muscle.

Difference Between Faradic and Galvanic Currents

Either faradic currents or galvanic currents are used for stimulating muscles. Their basic differences are detailed in Table 28.3.

Table 28.3: Difference between Faradic and galvanic currents

Features	*Faradic*	*Galvanic*
Definition	Faradic currents are short duration interrupted direct current of duration less than 10 milliseconds and frequency 50–100 Hertz.	Galvanic currents are long duration interrupted direct current of duration more than 10 milliseconds and frequency 30 Hertz.
Sensation	Pin prickling sensation.	Stabbing or burning sensation.
On innervated muscle	Tetanic contraction (slow contraction and slow relaxation).	Brisk contraction (immediate contraction and immediate relaxation).
On denervated muscle	Not tolerated by the patient.	Results in sluggish contraction or worm like contraction.

Difference Between Motor Unit and Motor Point

Their differences are detailed in Table 28.4.

Table 28.4: Difference between motor unit and motor point

Motor unit	*Motor point*
It is the unit formed by Anterior horn cell, Motor neurone and Muscle fiber it supplies (Fig. 28.1).	It is the point where nerve enters the muscle (Fig. 28.2). In stimulation maximum contraction can be achieved. If we place the pen electrode at motor point.

Motor point for a superficial muscle is at the junction of upper and middle one third of the belly of the muscle. Motor point for a deeply placed muscle is at the point where the muscle becomes superficial.

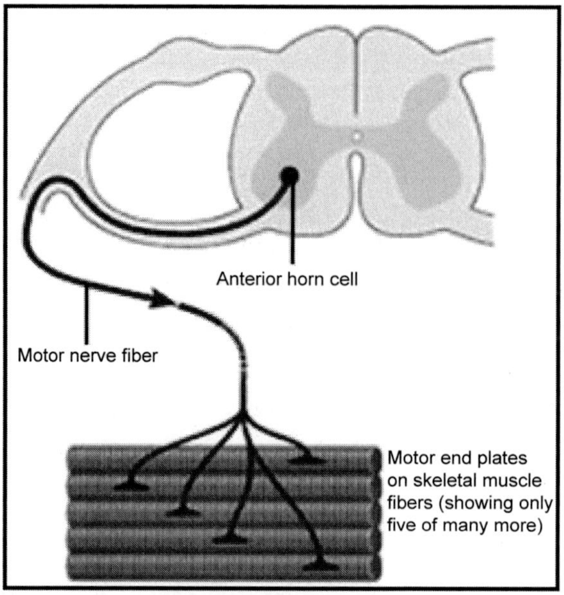

Fig. 28.1: Motor unit

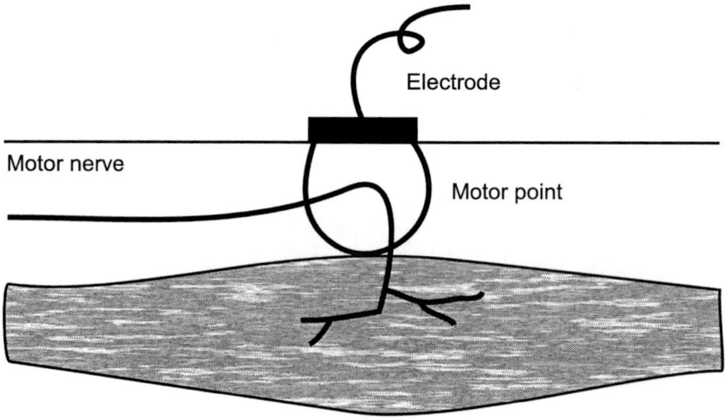

Fig. 28.2: Motor point

Electrode Orientation

To stimulate nerve, current must flow through tissue between two electrodes which are normally positioned so that current flows parallel to the nerve fibers (Fig. 28.3). If the current flow is at right angles to the fibers, much higher stimulus intensities are required (Fig. 28.4). If it is parallel to the nerve fiber greatest potential difference will be produced between adjacent nodes.

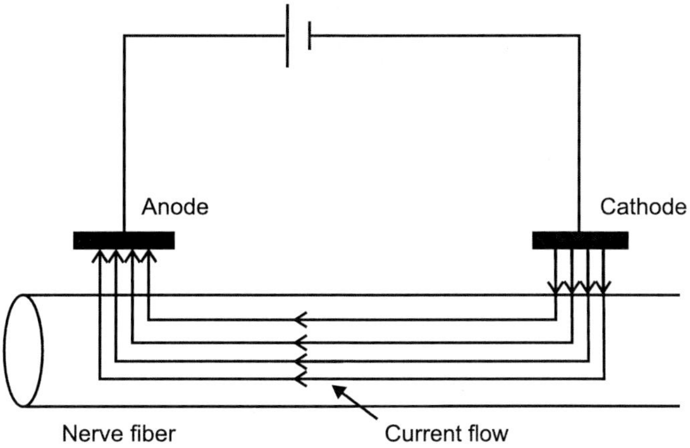

Fig. 28.3: Current flow parallel to nerve fiber

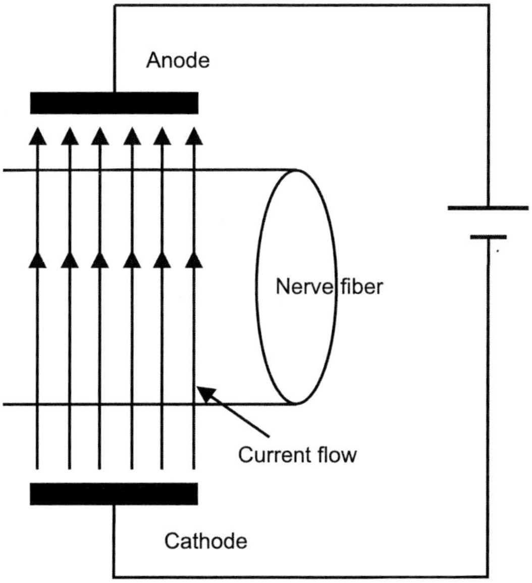

Fig. 28.4: Current flow perpendicular to nerve fiber

Effect of Stimulation Under Electrodes

At rest there is outside positive and inside negative. When a nerve is stimulated the current flows from negative to positive (Fig. 28.5).

Area Under Cathode

When a current is passed area under the cathode becomes negative so area under the cathode has maximal stimulation.

Area Under Anode

Electrons are moving away from the anode so area under the anode becomes more positive. There is a potential difference existing between area under the anode and adjacent area near the anode (Area under the anode is more positive and area nearby anode is less positive). Therefore, the adjacent area will be stimulated in case of anode.

In summary both anode and cathode can stimulate the nerve.

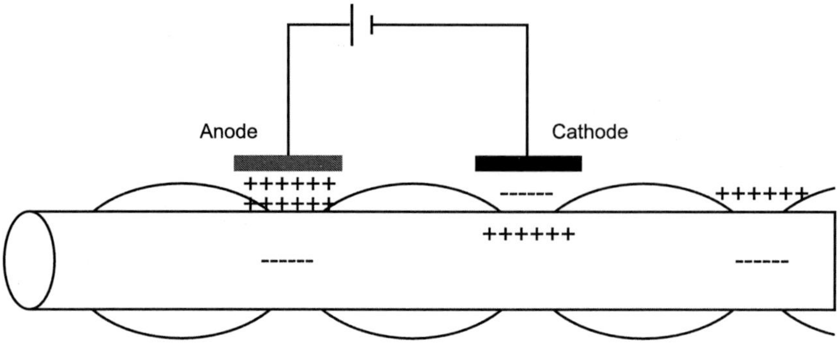

Fig. 28.5: Effects of stimulation under cathode and anode

Effect of Stimulation on Different Nerves

1. **Effect of stimulation in nerve trunk:** Stimulation of the middle of the nerve trunk results in generating impulse which goes to either side. Orthodromic impulses cross the synapse whereas antidromic conduction will not cross the first synapse (Figs. 28.6A and B).

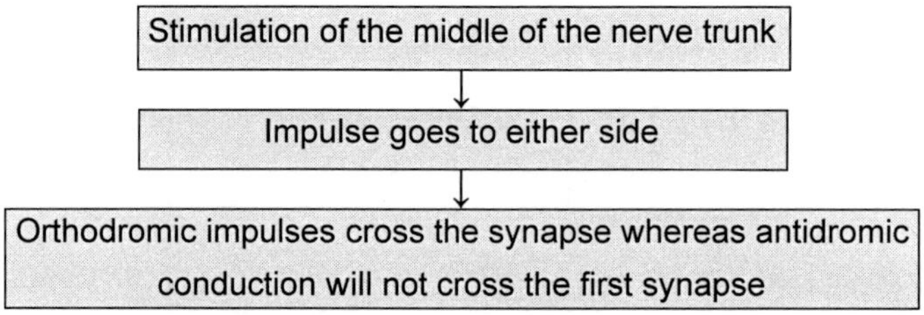

Fig. 28.6A: Effect of stimulation in nerve trunk

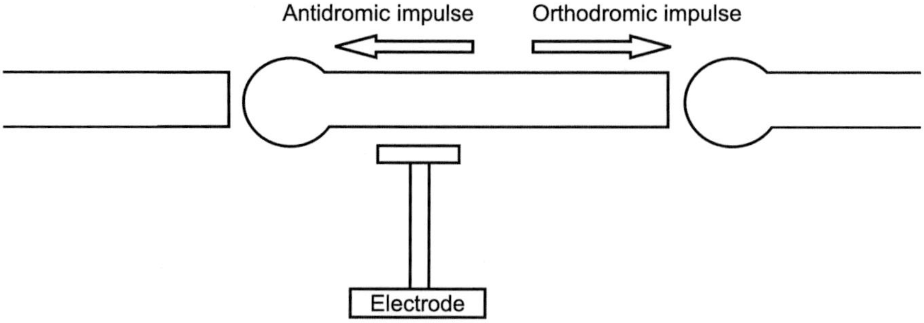

Fig. 28.6B: Effect of stimulation in nerve trunk

2. **Effect of stimulation on a motor nerve:** Upward travelling impulse will not cross first synapse whereas the downward travelling impulse reaches the muscle supplied to it to produce muscle contraction. Faradic current results in tetanic contraction and galvanic current results in brisk contraction if the muscle is innervated (Figs. 28.7A and B).

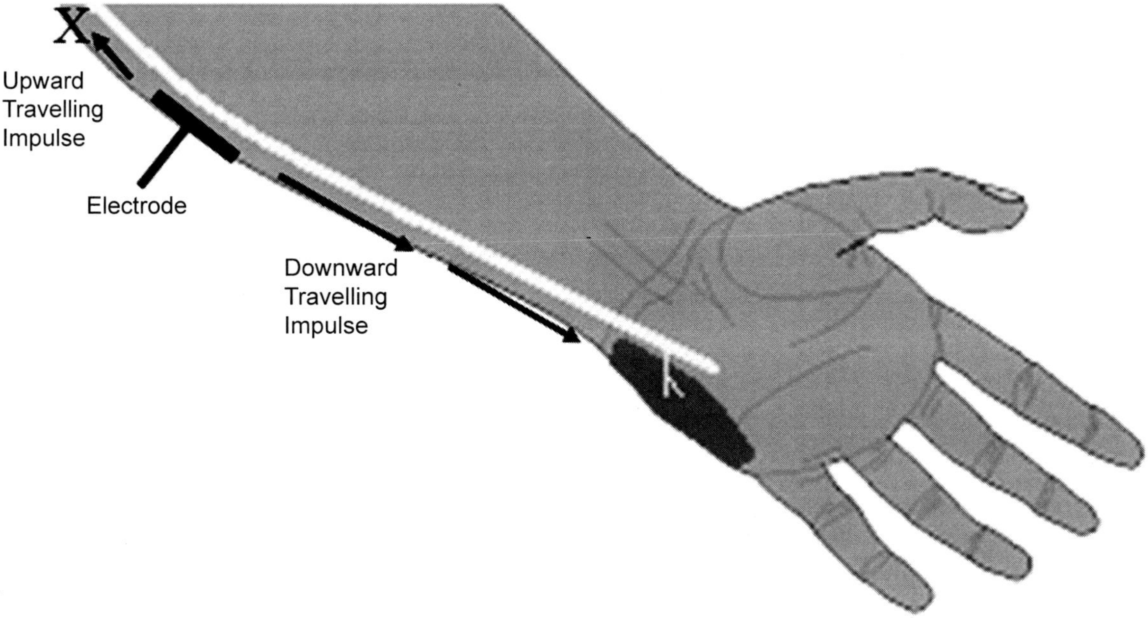

Fig. 28.7A: Effect of stimulation on a motor nerve

Stimulation of motor nerve

↓

Upward travelling impulse will not cross first synapse whereas the download travelling impulse reaches the muscle supplied

↓

Produces muscle contraction

↓

Faradic current results in tetanic contraction, galvanic current results in brisk contraction if the muscle is innervated

Fig. 28.7B: Effect of stimulation on a motor nerve

3. **Effect of stimulation on a sensory nerve:** Stimulation of a sensory nerve results in formation of two impulses. Downward travelling impulse does not have any effect (antidromic) whereas the upward travelling impulse reaches the spinal cord (orthodromic). Short duration faradic current results in pin prickling sensation whereas long duration galvanic current results in stabbing or burning sensation (Figs. 28.8A and B).

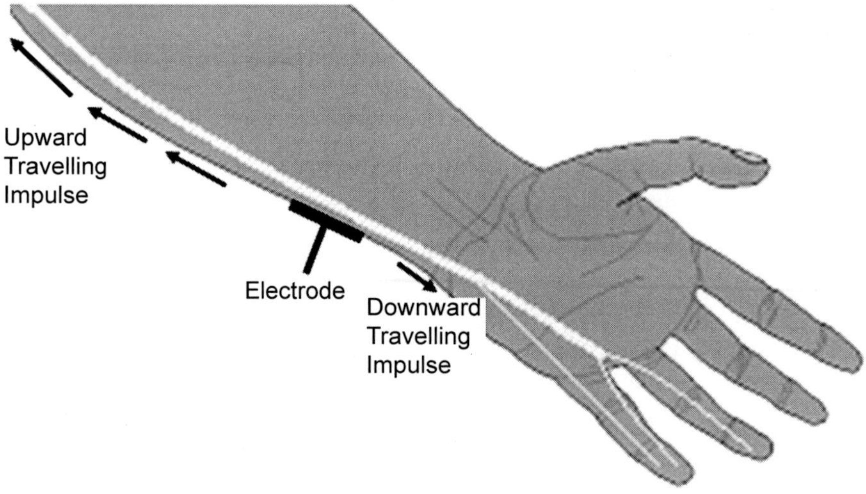

Fig. 28.8A: Effect of stimulation on a sensory nerve

Stimulation of a sensory nerve

↓

Download travelling impulse does not have any effect whereas the upward travelling impulse reaches the spinal cord (orthodromic)

↓

Pin prickling/burning sensation

Fig. 28.8B: Effect of stimulation on a sensory nerve

4. **Effect on stimulation of motor nerve trunk:** All the muscles that the nerve supplies below the point at which it is stimulated cause them to contract (Fig. 28.9).

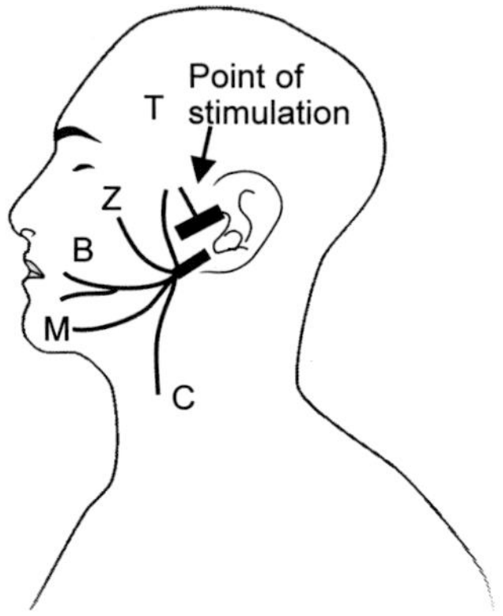

Branches of facial nerve: T = Temporal, Z = Zygomatic, B = Buccal, M = Mandibular, C = Cervical

Fig. 28.9: Effect on stimulation of facial motor nerve trunk

5. **Effect on stimulation of a motor point:** Stimulation of motor point results in maximum contraction than any other point (Fig. 28.10).

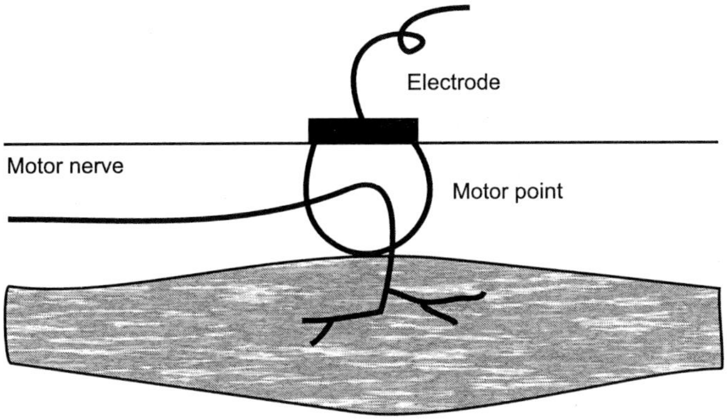

Fig. 28.10: Stimulation of a motor point

6. **Effect on mixed nerve:** Stimulation of mixed nerve results in muscle contraction and perceived sensation at same time.

Effect of Stimulation on the Strength of Muscle Contraction

It depends on the number of motor units recruited which in turn depends on the intensity of current applied and the rate of change of current. If the intensity of current rises suddenly there is no time for accommodation to take place which results in stronger muscle contraction. If the current rises slowly accommodation takes place than greater intensity is required produce same muscle contraction.

Effects of Frequency on Stimulation

When a single stimulus is applied there is sudden brisk contraction followed by immediate relaxation. (Isolated muscle contraction and the complete relaxation between the impulses). If the stimulation is given at the rate of 20 Hz, there is no time for complete relaxation which results in partial tetany. If the stimulation is above 60 Hz, there is no perceptible relation which results in full tetany (Fig. 28.11).

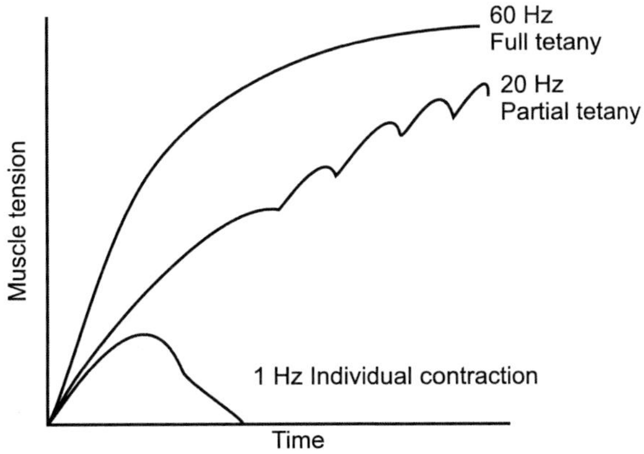

Fig. 28.11: Effects of frequency on stimulation

Effects of Pulse Duration on Stimulation

For an innervated muscle, for each of the long duration pulses same intensity is required to produce contraction and for each reduction in short duration pulses intensity has to be increased to produce same muscle contraction. For a denervated muscle, for each reduction in long duration pulses the intensity has to be increased to produce same muscle contraction. Short duration pulses will not be responded by a denervated muscle. The order of recruitment is usually sensory then motor then pain at all pulse durations when current is applied transcutaneously. The next important point is shorter the pulse duration the discrimination between sensory motor and pain response is also increased. This discrimination can be due to (1) fiber diameter, (2) depth of nerve fibers within the tissue and (3) electrical characteristics of nerve and skin.

1. **Fiber diameter:** Smaller the diameter of nerve fibers the larger is the chronaxie, larger is the associated time constant so long duration pulses can stimulate small diameter fibers with less intensity as compared to short duration pulses.
2. **Depth of the nerve fibers within the tissue:** As the depth increases the current is spreading and a consequent reduction in the local stimulus intensity. Superficially located fibers are therefore recruited at lower stimulus intensities.
3. **Electrical characteristics of nerve and skin:** The capacitive nature of the stratum corneum means that longer duration pulses are not more effective for nerve stimulation as current flow beneath skin reaches will be less.

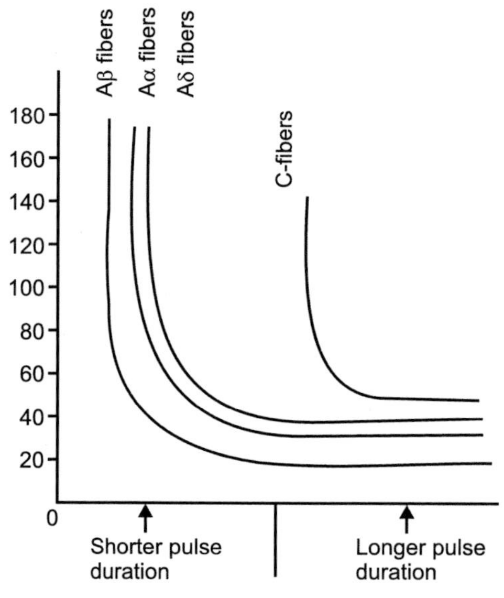

Fig. 28.12: Effects of pulse duration on stimulation

Hot Spot

Q. 1. Why galvanic currents (long duration pulses) are more painful compared to faradic currents (short duration pulses) in nerve-muscle stimulation?

Ans: With long duration pulses the ease of discrimination between C fiber and Aα is less. This results in activation of pain fibers which results in stabbing sensation with muscle contraction. Another reason is with long duration pulses most of the current is wasted in skin itself which activates C fibers.

Q. 2. How can we increase discrimination between sensory and motor response?

Ans: It depends on four factors:

Electrode placement: If electrodes are nearer to motor point; more motor response and if electrodes are far from motor point and nerve trunk; more sensory response.

Electrode size: If size is big more sensory stimulation, if size is less; more motor stimulation.

Pulse width: If pulse width is small better to discriminate sensory motor and pain response.

Stimulus frequency: 30 Hz painful muscle contraction, 50 Hz prickling muscle contraction.

29

Structure of Neuromuscular Electrical Stimulator/Neuromuscular Diagnostic Stimulator

TYPES OF STIMULATOR

There are several types of commercial classes of stimulator mentioned in the literature. It is detailed in Table 29.1.

Table 29.1: Types of stimulator and its goal

Type of electrical stimulation	*Goal*
Neuromuscular Diagnostic Stimulator (NMDS)	Cabinet type, used for diagnostic purpose, such as FG testing, For plotting SD curve and therapeutic for Nerve muscle stimulation and iontophoresis.
Neuromuscular Electrical Stimulation (NMES)	Cabinet type or portable, stimulation of innervated muscle to restore function including muscle strength, reduction of spasm/spasticity, prevention of atrophy, increase ROM, and muscle reeducation.
Electrical Muscle Stimulation (EMS)	Portable, stimulation of denervated muscle to maintain viability.
Electrical Stimulation for Tissue Repair (ESTR)	Portable or cabinet type, stimulation for edema reduction, increased circulation, and wound management
Functional Electrical Stimulation (FES)	Portable, neural implantation for long-term muscle activation to perform functional activities.
Transcutaneous Electrical Nerve Stimulation (TENS)	Portable, superficial stimulation across the skin for pain management.

INTERNAL FEATURE OF STIMULATOR

Each stimulator consists of step down transformer, rectifier, smoothing circuit, modulator circuit, oscillator circuit and amplifier (Fig. 29.1). Functions are mentioned below:

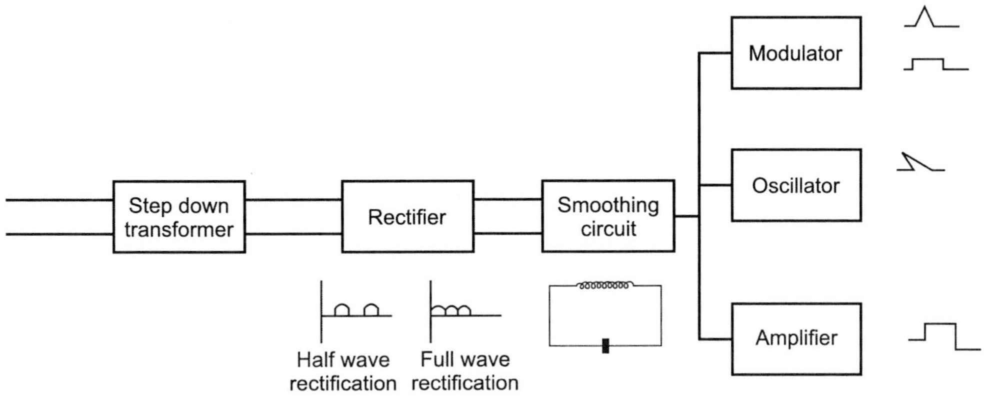

Fig. 29.1: Internal features of a stimulator

- Step down transformer: To reduce the voltage.
- Rectifier: Converts AC to DC.
- Smoothing circuit: Increases the current gradually with the help of inductor and to reduce the intensity gradually to the zero with the help of the capacitor.
- Modulator circuit: To determine the shape of current.
- Oscillator circuit: To determine the pulse duration, pulse interval and frequency.
- Amplifier circuit: Increases intensity of current.

EXTERNAL FEATURE OF STIMULATOR

Figure 29.2 shown below is a sample block diagram of neuromascular diagnostic stimulator. The knobs used in this type of stimulator are mentioned below:

1. On/Off switch.
2. Socket for connecting electrodes for faradic stimulation.
3. Socket for connecting electrodes for galvanic stimulation.
4. Switch to interchange between faradic and galvanic stimulation.
5. Pulse per second: Either one pulse in two seconds or one or two pulse in one second.
6. Display to show the intensity of galvanic stimulation.
7. Knob to select duration from 0.01 mS to 1000 mS or can put into G mode for iontophoresis.
8. Intensity knob of galvanic stimulation.
9. Knob for surging in faradic stimulation.
10. Intensity knob of faradic stimulation.

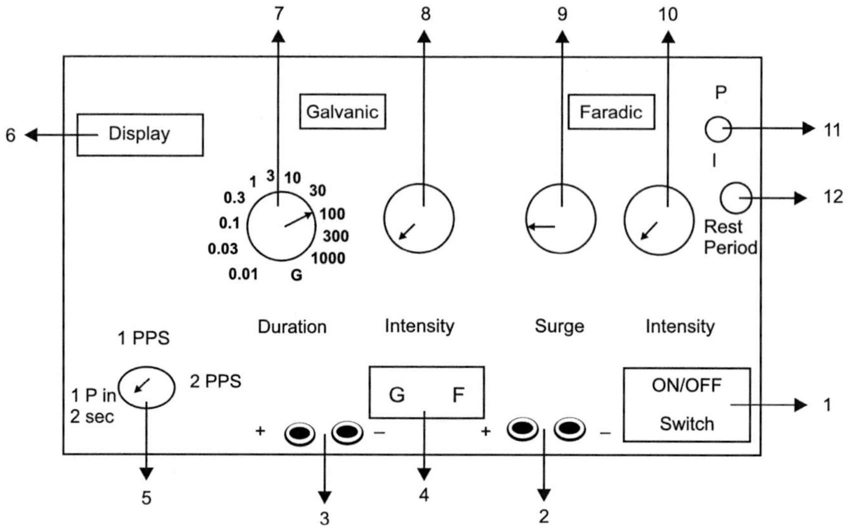

Fig. 29.2: External features of a stimulator

11. Knob to switch between plain faradic and intermittent faradic.
12. Knob for putting rest period between surges.

Knob 5, 7, 8 are used for galvanic stimulation and Knob 9, 10, 11, 12 are used for faradic stimulation.

CLASSIFICATION OF STIMULATOR

Stimulators can be classified based on their external power source (battery versus line power), based on display and setting the control knob (analog versus digital), based on the intention of use (therapeutic versus diagnostic) and by the nature of electrical stimulus, i.e., applied to the patient (constant current versus constant voltage). Advantages and disadvantages of each stimulator is described below:

1. **Line operated power stimulator**

   Advantages

   - Treatment can be given for longer period (stimulation parameters should remain at set levels for as long as the treatment is provided.
   - Many number of patients can be treated .
   - Higher amplitude can be achieved.

   Disadvantages

   - There is chance of shock.
   - Patient should remain stationary.
   - Apparatus is immobile or stationary, i.e., always near to the plug.

2. **Battery operated**

   Advantages

   - Small and portable.

- Stimulator is mobile, i.e., easily accessible to the patient.
- The client can move (during ambulation, stimulation of pain control while a patient is on the job.
- Less shock.

Disadvantages

- Short battery life.
- Lower amplitude.

3. **Analog stimulator**

Advantages

- Ability to continuously adjust many of the stimulation parameters.
- Less time consuming.

Disadvantages

- Not pre-programmed.
- More knobs to control the setting.

4. **Digital stimulator**

Advantages

- Pre-programmed.
- Less knobs to control the setting.

Disadvantages

- More time consuming.
- Only intensity parameter can be increased.
- User has to scroll for menu.

5. **Therapeutic stimulator**

Advantages

- Portable.
- Treatment can be carried by the patient.
- Not painful to the patient.

Disadvantages

- Less number of knobs to control the treatment parameter hence, cannot be used during stages of denervation and reinnervation.
- Less number of knob to control the settings.

6. **Diagnostic stimulator**

Advantages

- The patient can be treated stages of denervation and reinnervation.
- More number of knobs to control the setting.

Disadvantages

- More painful
- Machine is immobile

7. **Constant current; and**
8. **Constant voltage stimulator.**

Stimulators can be constant current or constant voltage based on the nature of electrical stimulus, i.e., applied to the patient. They cannot be both at the same time. According to Ohm's law (V/I = R) if voltage is kept constant and skin resistance is increased, the current delivered to the tissue is reduced. If current is kept constant if skin resistance is increased voltage will be increased to deliver the same current.

Constant Current Stimulators produce a constant current independent of resistance encountered. The voltage adjusts to maintain constant current flow. The advantage of this type of stimulator is to ensure a consistency physiologic response during the treatment. The negative is potential pain when the voltage increases to overcome resistance.

Constant Voltage Stimulators, conversely, produce a constant voltage. The current adjusts to depending on changes in resistance. This unit is advantageous in preventing discomfort with changes in resistance, such as an electrode losing full contact, but quality of response can be decreased with these automatic resistance changes.

Advantages and disadvantages of these stimulators are listed in Table 29.2. The electrode events and its effects on constant current and constant voltage is listed in Table 29.3.

To determine constant current versus constant voltage on an electrical stimulation unit, slowly start to peel one electrode off the skin while the machine is on. If the current sharpens, the machine is constant current; if the current lessens, the machine is constant voltage when the electrode is being peeled away.

Table 29.2: Constant current versus constant voltage stimulator

Device	*Constant current*	*Constant voltage*
Advantage	Automatically reduces the driving voltage when electrode contact improve as electrical transmission increases	When the contact is reduced it reduces the current, it results in less burns
Disadvantage	When electrode contact reduces constant current stimulator increases the driving voltage which results in burns	If contact is more it results in high level of stimulation, the patient cannot tolerate

Table 29.3: Electrode events and its effects on types of stimulator

Event	*Change in impedance*	*Effect if constant current*	*Effect if constant voltage*
Electrodes drying on skin	Increase	No effect	Reduced current
Electrodes pushed against skin	Decrease	No effect	Increased current
Electrode lifting off skin	Increase	Increase current density	Reduced current
Increased sweating under electrode	Decrease	No effect	Increased current and current density

CURRENT WAVEFORM

Definition: The geometric or the graphical description of the shape, direction, amplitude, duration, and pulse frequency of a DC, AC, pulsed DC or pulsed AC currents.

Types

1. **Monophasic:** A pulse that moves in only one direction either + or – e.g., DC currents.
2. **Biphasic:** A pulse that moves in both directions, e.g., AC currents.
   It can be of following types:
   (a) *Symmetrical:* A biphasic pulse with both phases geometrically equal to each other.
   (b) *Asymmetrical:* A biphasic pulse with both phases geometrically different to each other.
   (c) *Balanced:* A biphasic pulse with equal electrical charges in each phase.
   (d) *Unbalanced:* A biphasic pulse with unequal electrical charges in each phase.

   Symmetrical pulses are always balanced whereas asymmetrical waveforms are either balanced or unbalanced.
3. *Polyphasic:* Bidirectional wave with three or more phases in bursts. All polyphasic pulses are bursts but not all bursts are polyphasic.

   Please see Figure 29.3 for different types of waveforms.

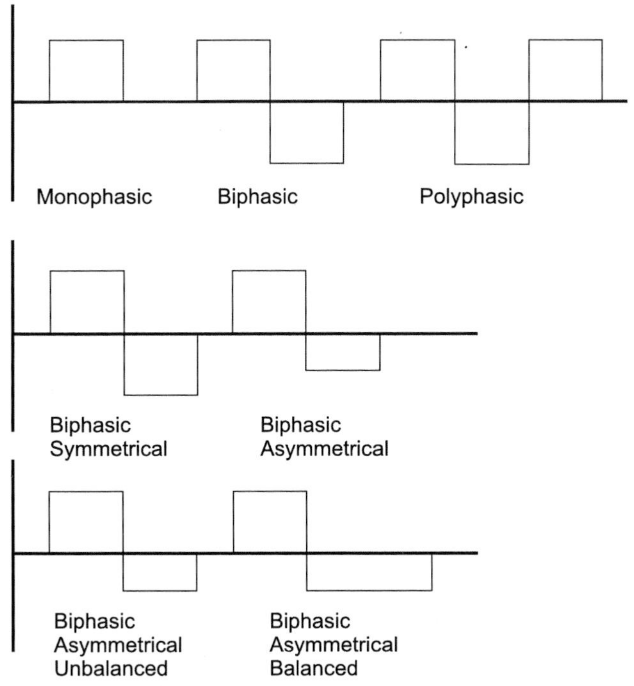

Fig. 29.3: Types of waveforms

Waveform Selection

- All waveforms are capable of activating peripheral nerves.
- Symmetrical biphasic waveforms pose the least risk for skin reaction.
- Monophasic waveforms are most appropriate for wound healing.
- Asymmetrical balanced biphasic waveforms may be more useful to stimulate small muscle groups.
- Monophasic and symmetrical biphasic waveforms generate greater torque with muscle contraction and were less fatiguing than polyphasic waveforms.

Hot Spot

Cycle applies to biphasic current whereas pulse applies to monophasic currents.

SHAPE

Electrical currents may take sinusoidal, rectangular, square, trapezoidal, saw tooth or spiked configuration. In this rectangular and square shaped pulses are fast rising pulses (Fig. 29.4). They are used for stimulation of innervated muscles. Triangular, trapezoidal, saw tooth and depolarized pulses are called as slow rising pulses or selective pulses or accommodation pulses (Fig. 29.5). They are preferred for the stimulation of denervated muscle. Since nerve has the property of accommodation, slow rising pulses are not used for the stimulation of innervated muscle.

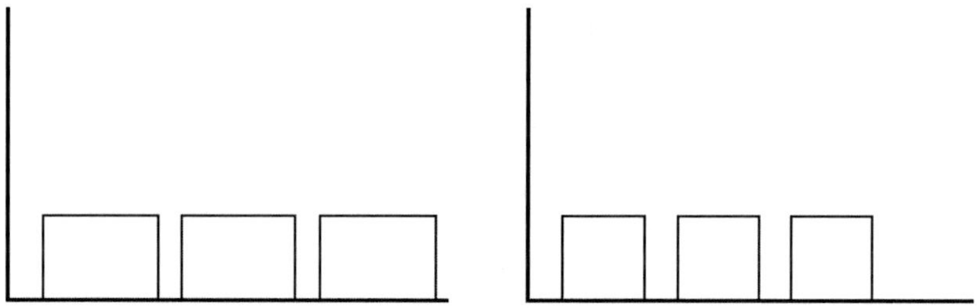

(a) Rectangular (b) Square

Fig. 29.4: Fast rising pulses

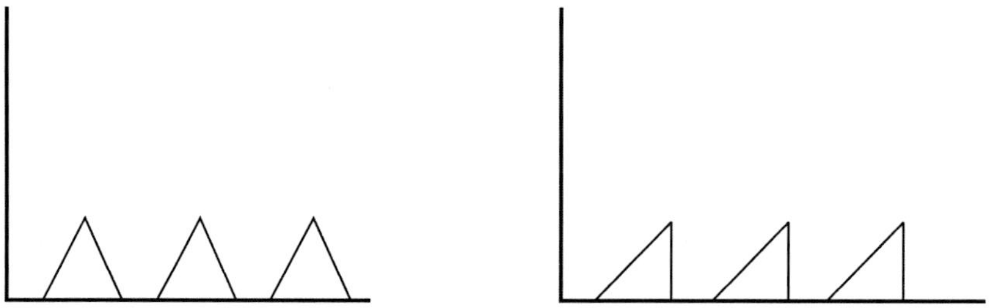

(a) Triangular (b) Saw tooth

Contd.

Contd.

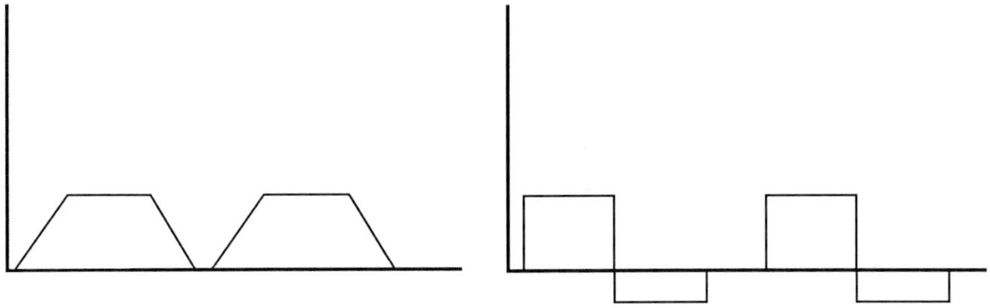

(c) Trapezoidal (d) Depolarized

Fig. 29.5: Slow rising pulses

Hot Spot

Selective pulses (accommodation pulses)
The impulse in which the current rises gradually is called as selective pulses.
Types:
1. Saw tooth
2. Trapezoid
3. Triangular
4. Depolarized pulse
Uses: Used in the stimulation of denervated muscle.

Depolarized Pulse

Some equipment allows a low intensity reverse current between the impulse and so called pulses are depolarized pulse (Fig. 29.5). The reversed wave of current between the impulses reduces the chemical formation. The quantity of electricity passed in the reverse current is equal to than in the forward one any chemical forms are neutralized and danger of burn is eliminated.

DURATION (Fig. 29.6)

(a) *Phase duration:* The time that each pulse lasts is called the phase duration.

(b) *Pulse duration or pulse width:* The time elapsed from the beginning to the end of the two phases within a pulse or cycle including the interphase duration if present (sum of all phases + interphase or intrapulse duration).

(c) *Interpulse duration:* The time elapsed between two successive pulses or cycles.

(d) *Burst duration:* The time elapsed between the beginning of the first and end of the last pulse within each burst (Burst is defined as an interrupted train of pulses).

(e) *Interburst duration:* The time elapsed between two successive bursts.

FREQUENCY

Frequency is the number of times per second that a pulse, cycle, burst or beat will repeat itself.

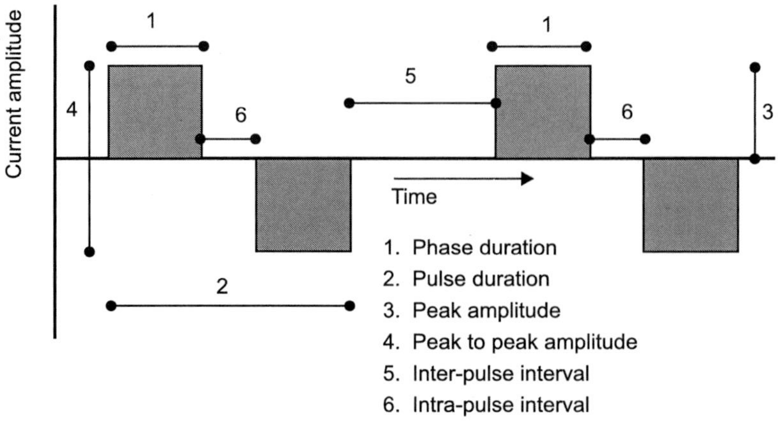

Fig. 29.6: Different terminologies of duration

Types

(a) *Pulse frequency:* The number of pulses per second (pps).

(b) *Cycle frequency:* The number of cycles per second (cps or Hz).

(c) *Burst frequency:* The number of bursts per second (bups).

(d) *Beat frequency:* The number of beats per second (beps). It is determined by the difference between frequencies of both channels in IFT.

AMPLITUDE

Amplitude is the magnitude of current being the tip relative to the isoelectric (zero) baseline, expressed in μA or mA. It is synonymous with the terms voltage and current intensity.

Types

(a) *Peak amplitude:* The maximum amplitude of one or more phases relative to the zero baseline.

(b) *Average amplitude:* The mean current amplitude applied to the tissues over the waveform period.

(c) *Root mean square amplitude:* The total effective current acting on the tissues over a period of time.

MODULATION

It refers to any alteration in the amplitude, duration, or frequency of the current during a series of pulses or cycles.

Types

1. *Continuous current:* The amplitude of the current flow remains same for several seconds to minute, e.g., Iontophoresis.
2. *Burst modulation:* It occurs when current flows for a short duration and turned off for a short time in a repetitive cycle, e.g., Russian currents, Burst TENS.

3. *Beat modulation:* It will be produced when interference of two biphasic currents delivered separately through different channels. This produces a beat frequency which is equal to difference in frequency between the biphasic current frequencies, e.g., IFT.
4. *Ramping or surging modulation:* The current amplitude will increase gradually to preset maximum and may also decrease suddenly or gradually down in intensity, e.g., surged faradism (Fig. 29.7).

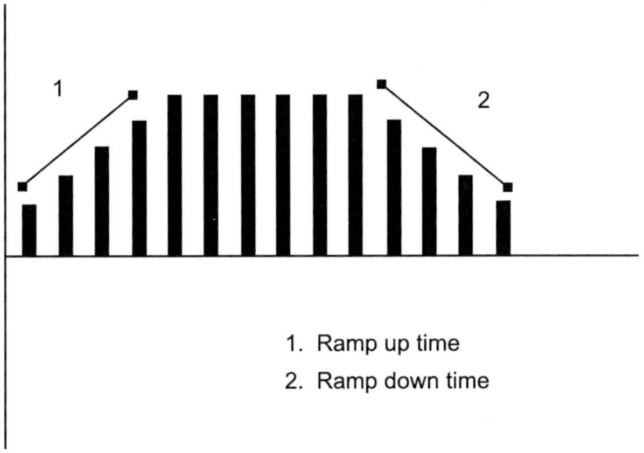

Fig. 29.7: Ramping

OTHER TERMINOLOGIES

- *On time:* The period of time the current is on for particular duration during which the stimulator delivers the current into the tissues.
- *Off time:* The period of time during which the stimulator delivers no current to the tissues.
- *Duty cycle:* It is the ratio of on time to the summation of on time plus off time and expressed as percentage.
- *Ramp up time:* The time elapsed from the onset or baseline to plateau current amplitude or maximum of the train or the time taken to reach the peak current (Fig. 29.7).
- *Ramp down time:* The time elapsed from the plateau current amplitude to zero baseline (Fig. 29.7).
- *Phase rise time:* Time takes for the leading edge of any one phase to rise from zero baseline to its maximum amplitude.
- *Phase decay time:* The time it takes for the trailing edge of any one phase to decay from maximum amplitude to the zero baseline.

Phase rise or decay time happens only during a phase. This is different from ramp up or ramp down time.

30

Principles of Application

ELECTRODE TISSUE INTERFACE

It is the junction of electrode with that of skin separated by a coupling medium. Coupling medium may be an electrode gel (Fig. 30.1) or lint pad soaked in water (Fig. 30.2). Electrochemical changes takes place at this junction. If applied current is evenly alternating current or biphasic pulse, there will be no chemical changes take place. If applied current is unidirectional with high intensity, chemical changes can take place.

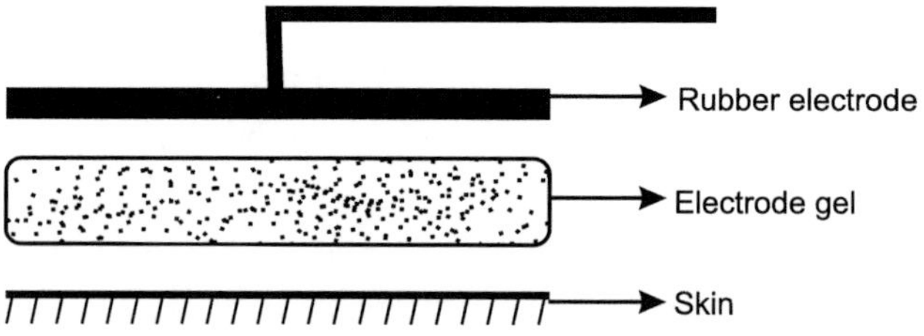

Fig. 30.1: Electrode tissue interface with electrode gel

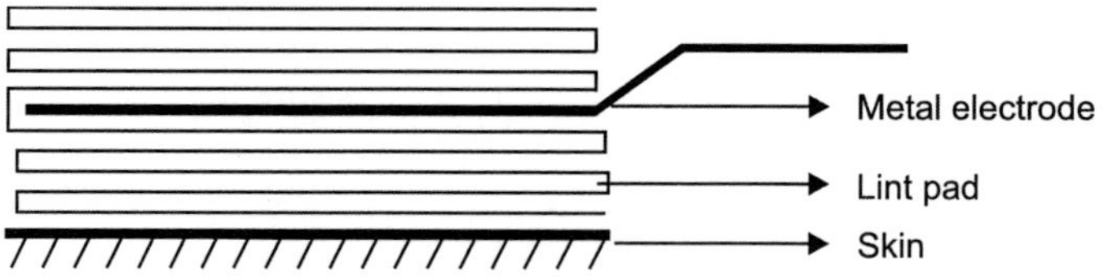

Fig. 30.2: Electrode tissue interface with lint pad

ELECTRODE COUPLING MEDIA

Definition

The material which is added between the skin and electrode is coupling media.

Types

It can be of any of the following:

- Electrode gel (made up of ionic salts) (NaCl, KCl), water, surfactant, fungicide and bactericide.
- Lint pad which is soaked in water.
- Sponge soaked in water.
- Pen electrode soaked in water.
- Self adhesive gel.

Purpose

- To pass the current from electrode to the skin so that uniform conducting pathway exists between electrode and skin.
- To make electrode chemical changes occur outside the skin.
- To reduce skin resistance (skin resistance is due to a protein called keratin, dry scaly skin or due to presence of sebum).

ELECTRODE

Definition

Electrode represents the instrument for current delivery from electric stimulator to skin.

Classification

Electrodes are classified mainly on its purpose, function and shape.

1. Classification based on its purpose:
   (a) Surface electrode is used for NMES (Neuromuscular electric stimulator)
   (b) Needle electrode used for recording the EMG.
2. Classification of surface electrode:
   (a) Metal electrode
   (b) Carbon impregnated rubber electrode
   (c) Self adhesive single use electrode
   (d) Self adhesive reusable electrode.
3. Classification of needle electrodes:
   (a) Concentric
   (b) Single needle
4. Classification of electrodes based on shape:
   (a) Rectangular electrode
   (b) Circular electrode
   (c) Pen electrode

(d) Butterfly electrode (used in TENS)
(e) Disc electrode
(f) Button electrode
(g) Ring electrode.

5. Classification of electrode based on function:
(a) Active electrode
(b) Inactive electrode
(c) Ground electrode
(d) Recording electrode
(e) Reference electrode.

6. Electrode used for prosthesis:
(a) Textile electrode
(b) Array electrode.

Description of Electrodes

Only some electrodes are described here.

A. Metal electrode

Combination: Made up of metal plate of either tin, steel, aluminium or zinc.

Advantages:

- High conductivity
- Long lasting or durable.

Disadvantages:

- Not flexible
- Less likely to mould towards the skin counter
- Chance of getting shock
- Difficulty to secure comfortably
- Few size of electrode availability.

Coupling media:

- 16 layers of lint pad with water or cotton with water
- Wet sponge
- Artificial sponge material called spontex.

Binding: With the help of strap or body weight.

B. Carbon impregnated rubber electrode

Combination: Rubber with silicon or carbon polymer.

Advantages:

- Flexible

- Less chance of shock
- More likely to mould on the skin
- Treatment of deeper areas.

Disadvantages:

- It is not long lasting
- Presence of hot spot
- No uniform current delivery
- Less conduction.

Coupling media: Electrode gel.

Binding: Straps, Micro pore tapes, Body weight, Plaster.

C. Self adhesive electrode

Combination: It is made up of rubber with silicon or carbon polymer with self adhesive gel.

Advantages:

- No strapping or taping is required.

Disadvantages:

- For single used electrode: It is costly
- For reuse electrode: It produces cross contamination.

Coupling media: Synthetic gel, karaya gel.

Binding: No binding is required.

D. Pen electrode:

Description: These are the rounded metal head covered with cotton and again covered with lint.

Advantages:

- Stimulation
- Used for diagnostic purpose
- Mobile
- Less chance of burn
- Long lasting
- Good conduction
- Stimulation of small muscle
- Stimulation of individual muscle.

Disadvantages:

- Holding the electrode for long time (tiredness to physiotherapist)
- Periodic soaking is necessary
- Depending on pressure, current delivered will increase or decrease
- Cannot stimulate deep seated muscle.

Coupling media: water (period soaking).

Binding: Holding the electrode in the hand.

TISSUE IMPEDANCE

The quantity and the path of the current flowing in the tissue depend on the impedance of the pathway. Electrical current applied to the body through surface, electrodes and encounters resistance at two types of electrodes skin interface. Tissue impedance is the sum of these Ohmic resistance and capacitive resistance. Inductive resistance does not influence the effects of electrical stimulation.

Ohmic resistance: Ohmic resistance depends on electrode surface area; inter electrode distance, skin temperature, dryness (due to keratin), thickness and nature of skin, the amount of skin oil (sebum) and presence of hair. Ohmic resistance is inversely proportional to size of electrodes but directly proportional to dryness of skin, to hairy skin. Clipping excessive hair increases electrode surface area. However, following these preparations skin resistance often remains relatively high.

Capacitive resistance: Capacitive resistance occurs where an electrode is separated from the nerve and muscle by skin and fat. When current is applied to skin there is also presence of a capacitive resistance, i.e., inversely related to pulse frequency. Electric current perfuse through tissues creates a force on electrically charged ions present at interfaces between different types of tissues and in cell membranes. The conduction of current through tissues depends on ionic movement. When electrical current are introduced into the body ions accumulate at tissues interfaces and at cell membranes creating a charge, i.e., opposite to charge of voltage applied at electrodes. The potential difference that occurs between each electrode and tissues is created by electrolyte polarization. The counter voltage is called reactance or capacitance. As the frequency of biphasic pulse is increased pronounced decreased in capacitive skin resistance occurs.

The relationship of impedance with Frequency and Capacitance is as follows:

$$\text{Impedance} = \frac{1}{2\pi FC}$$

Z = Capacitive resistance or impedance.

F = Frequency in Hz

C = Capacitance of skin resistance.

Capacitance of skin cannot be changed.

Skin impedance is inversely proportional to frequency and capacitance of skin.

Electrical currents tend to choose the path that offers the least resistance to flow. The conductivity can be affected by tissue type and tissue health.

1. **Tissue Type:** Tissue impedance and conductivity vary through the body tissues depending on water content.
   (a) High water content decreases impedance and increased conductivity: Deeper layers of the skin, nerve and muscle.
   (b) Low water content increases impedance: Bone, fat, tendon, and fascia are poor conductors due to low water content, also the outer layer of the skin called epidermis.
2. **Tissue Health:** Tissue health will change impedance.
   (a) Impedance increases with edema, ischemia, atherosclerosis, scarring and denervation.
   (b) Impedance decreases with open wounds and abrasions.

So, the tissue with highest in water content and ion content will be the best conductor of electricity.

METHOD OF REDUCING SKIN RESISTANCE

A. **Washing:** To remove keratin and dead cell.

B. **Warming:** Increases rate of particle movement and ionic movement. It also increases activity of sweat glands. Warming can be done with hot packs or IRR prior to the treatment.

C. **Wetting:** Increases ionic movement.

D. **Scrapping:** Removes the dead cells from the outer epidermis. It remove sore of keratin and sebum.

WATER BATH

Definition

The technique consists of immersing a body part (hand and foot) in a bowel of water with the electrode dipped. This technique is used in treatment of hand, forearm, foot and leg.

Types

Bipolar Bath

If both electrodes are on same bath, it is referred to as bipolar bath. Here, current will pass through the water and through the tissue simultaneously. Thus, two pathways are in parallel. Adding salt to the bipolar bath will decrease current through the tissue since greater current is passed through parallel water pathway due to lower resistance. Bipolar bath is used for faradic foot bath in case of flat foot, hallux valgus and metatarsalgia (Fig. 30.3).

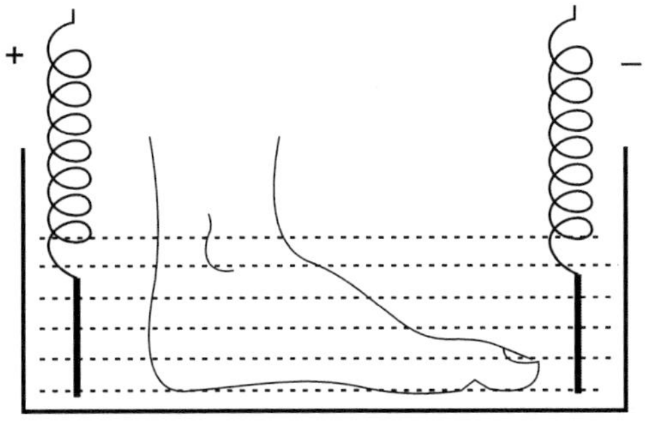

Fig. 30.3: Bipolar bath

Unipolar Bath

If one electrode is in bath and circuit is completed by pad electrode or an electrode in another bath refers to unipolar bath. Here, current first pass through water and then through tissue to complete circuit. Thus, two pathways are in series. Adding salt to a unipolar bath results in greater current passing through the tissues because it lowers resistance in series, thus, reducing the total resistance. Unipolar bath is used in case of hyperhydrosis or in case of iontophoresis application (Fig. 30.4).

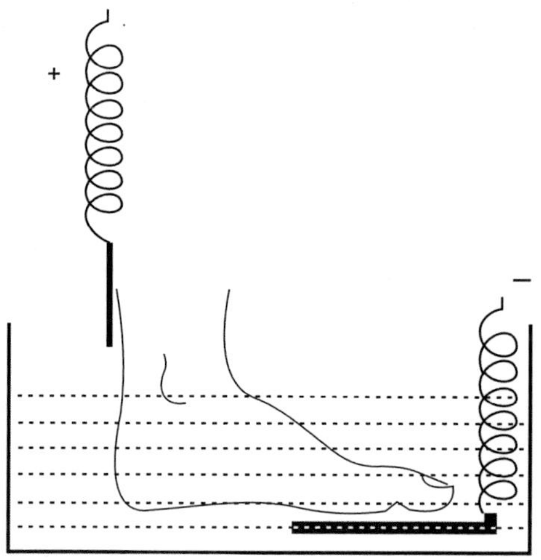

Fig. 30.4: Unipolar bath

CURRENT DENSITY

Amount of current flow per cubic volume is called as current density. It should be high enough to cause depolarization. The current density is highest where the electrodes meet the skin and diminishes as the electricity penetrates into deeper tissues.

Factors that Determines Current Density

- Interelectrode distance
- Electrode size.

Interelectrode Distance

The distance between electrodes is termed Interelectrode distance. If the electrodes are spaced closely together, the effect will be localized to the region between electrodes. The area of highest current density is relatively superficial. Hence, greater current is passed through the skin rather than through deep tissues. This increases the chance of burning the patient. If the electrodes are spaced farther apart, current density will be higher in the deeper tissues including nerve and the muscle. With wider spacing, greater current amplitude can often be used to reach the deeper tissues. Wider spacing can also lead to more motor units being activated (for an NMES application) or more sensory fibers activated (in a TENS mode) (Fig. 30.5).

Electrode Size

As the size of one electrode relative to another is decreased, the current density beneath the electrode is increased. The larger electrode has larger surface area so least current density. Smaller electrode produces high current density and it is used to stimulate motor point or for acupuncture point. Hence, small electrode is used as active electrode. The larger electrodes are more comfortable, greater level

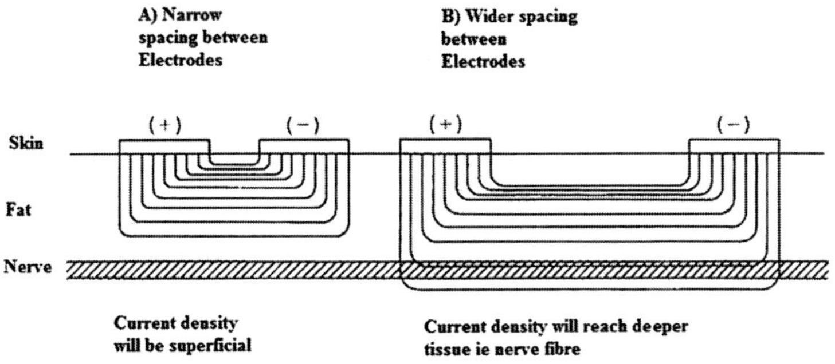

Fig. 30.5: Unequal current density; more at superficial

of sensory stimulation and have least current density. Inactive electrode should be far from electric stimulation and also should be large so less local effect\produces under inactive electrode. If electrodes are of same size the current density in each will be similar. So, this is used for group muscle stimulation and sensory stimulation in case of pain relief (Fig. 30.6).

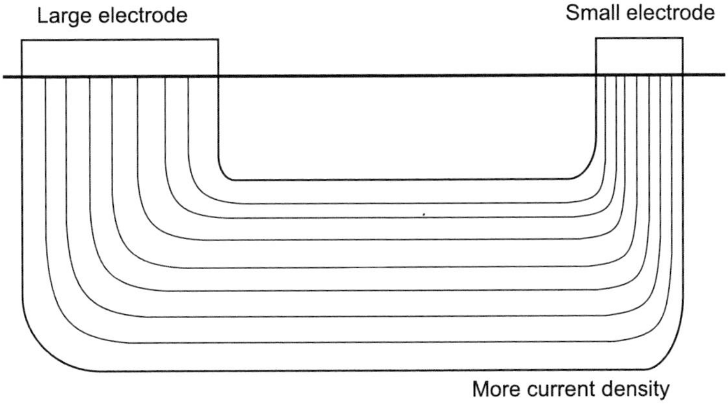

Fig. 30.6: More current density at smaller electrode

Factors which Determine the Size of Electrode

Skin impedance: Smaller electrode has higher impedance and less penetration whereas bigger electrode has less impedance and good penetration.

Pulse duration: More the pulse duration, more the impedance thus, less penetration.

Current density: Smaller electrode has more current density and more perception of current.

Specificity of stimulation: For motor point use pen electrode and for group muscle stimulation use rubber electrode or metal electrode.

Size of electrode: Smaller electrode results in muscle stimulation with pain whereas larger electrode results in muscle stimulation without pain.

Perceived discrimination of excitatory response: If it is for sensory purpose use larger electrode and smaller one for muscle stimulation.

POLARITY TESTING

There are three tests to check the polarity of electrodes. Any of the technique can be used:

1. The chemical changes which occur when a D.C. is passed through an electrolyte are used in determining the polarity of a direct current source of supply. If the bare ends of two leads connected to such a supply are placed in tap-water and the current turned on, bubbles of hydrogen gas appear round the negative wire.
2. In case of phenolphthalein experiment, add few drops of phenolphthalein over tissue paper and place the electrodes connected to direct current source over it, then pass the current for some time and then you will see pink color under negative electrode or cathode.
3. Alternatively litmus paper can be used. This is damped with tap-water and bare ends of the two leads from the source of current are pressed firmly on the paper about one inch apart. On the passage of current, blue litmus paper turns red with the acid at the anode, while red litmus paper turns blue with the alkali formed at the cathode.

In modern stimulators, the polarity is marked with "–" as cathode and "+" as anode. In the lead wires, the color coding is also used with black as cathode and red as anode. Since polarity is already marked in modern stimulators, nowadays polarity testing is not performed.

LAW OF POLAR EXCITATION (PFLUGER LAW)

A given segment of a nerve is irritated by the development of catelectrotonus and the disappearance of anelectrotonus, but the reverse does not hold; that is, excitation occurs at the cathode when the circuit is closed and at the anode when it is opened.

Muscle contraction can be produced during the break and make of the circuit (make means circuit is on or closed; break means circuit is off or open). When the circuit is on, area under the cathode action potential is produced and it is called cathode closing contraction (CCC).When the circuit is on, area adjacent to the anode action potential is produced and it is called Anode Closing contraction (ACC). When the circuit is off area under the anode, there is sudden loss of positive charge. This can produce action potential which is called anode opening contraction (AOC). When the circuit is off area adjacent to the cathode, action potential is produced which is called as cathode opening contraction (COC).

Polar Formula

It is also known as Erb's polar formula. The relationship between anodal and cathodal opening and closing currents has been called Erb's polar formulae. For a innervated muscle, the normal response obtained to cathode and anode is CCC>ACC>AOC>COC. Here CCC stands for cathodal closing current, ACC for anodal closing current, AOC for anodal opening current and COC for cathodal opening current. It means normally a better contraction is obtained with cathodal closing current than anodal closing current in a innervated muscle. Closing and opening terminologies are used because when this experiment must have been tried at that time simple key switch which is on by closing and off by opening must have been used. In denervation reversal of this formula may be noted. In denervated muscle, it may be ACC>CCC>COC>AOC. With the very short duration pulses used in modern stimulators, muscle contractions are not elicited by opening current stimulation. So, in denervated muscle either anode or cathode can be used as active electrode. It is concluded that when faradic currents are used active electrode is cathode and when galvanic currents are used either cathode or anode can be the active electrode.

ARRANGEMENT OR PLACEMENT OR CONFIGURATION OF ELECTRODE

The arrangement of electrode will greatly impact the effect of electrical stimulation. There are three basic techniques of electrode placement: (1) Monopolar, (2) Bipolar, (3) Quadripolar. The monopolar and bipolar methods can be simple or bifurcated. Bifurcation of lead wires can allow a greater area to be treated but decreases the current density at each individual electrode since the current is now shared between the electrodes (Fig. 30.7).

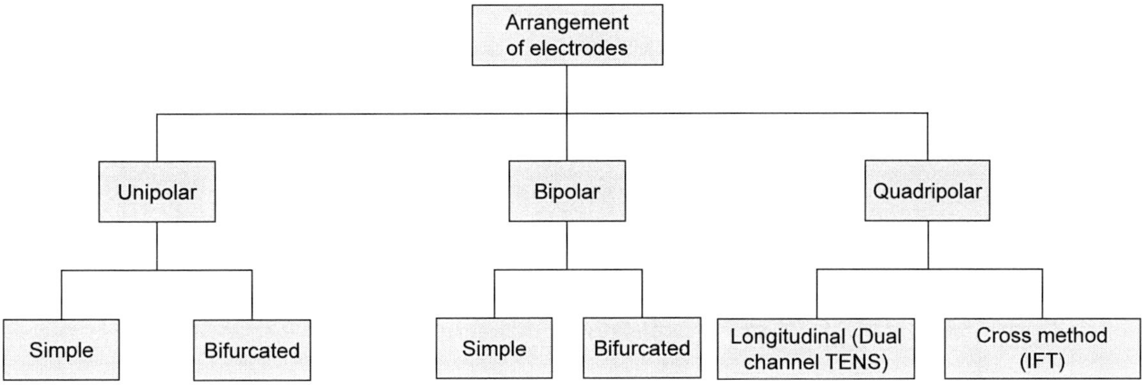

Fig. 30.7: Arrangement of electrodes

Monopolar (Unipolar)

When one electrode is placed on the target area it is called as monopolar technique. The other electrode is placed in the area that is not affected by stimulation. In this technique, one electrode is more active than the other electrode. Monopolar technique is used in case of dermal ulcer, wound, localized edema, trigger point, acupuncture point, iontophoresis and motor point area. This technique is used to stimulate a specific muscle belly. The electrode can be a button electrode or a pen electrode. The indifferent electrode is usually applied away from the muscle being stimulated. Limitations of unipolar electrode setup include problem with stimulating a muscle when the nerve trunk cannot be accessed. The total area of active treatment electrode should be less than the non-treatment electrode otherwise non-treatment electrode become active because of higher current density under that electrode. It can be simple or bifurcated. A simple method is used for stimulation of motor point and bifurcated method for the treatment of compartment (Fig. 30.8).

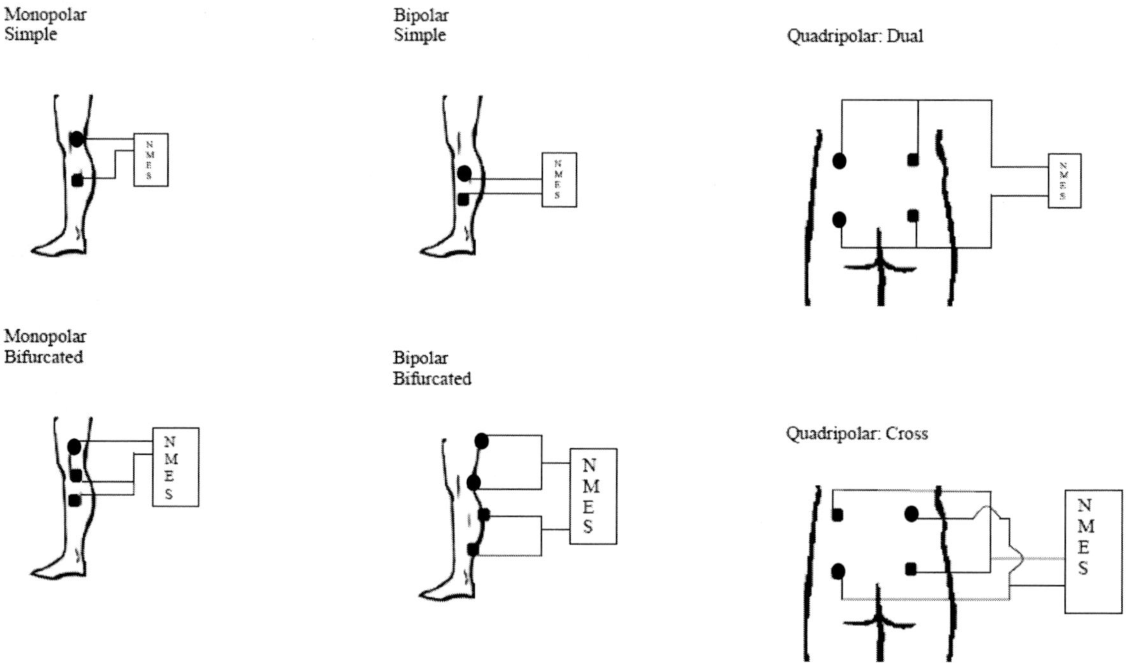

Fig. 30.8: Electrode

Bipolar

In this placement, all the electrodes of a single circuit are placed over the treatment area. A bipolar method uses two equal or nearly equal size electrodes placed at either end of the muscle belly or group to be stimulated. The current density will be equal under both electrodes. Bipolar placement is commonly preferred for denervated muscles. It can be simple or bifurcated. Simple is commonly preferred for group muscle stimulation (NMES and FES). Bifurcated is preferred in case of radiating pain or during faradism under pressure (Fig. 30.8).

Quadripolar

In these four electrodes are used which comes from two leads. This leads can be two channels from same stimulator or different stimulator. Two different types are used; longitudinal and crossed method. Longitudinal is used to treat large areas especially in case of painful area method of TENS application. One channel is put above the site of pain and other channel is put below the site of pain. In Crossed method commonly used with IFT where channel 1 and 2 are crossed each other so that effect will be more in the center where they cross (Fig. 30.8).

The treatment goal, condition used, position of electrodes and arrangement of electrodes are detailed in Table 30.1.

Table 30.1: Position and arrangement of elctrodes

Treatment goal	***Condition***	***Leads and electrodes***	***Monopolar***	***Bipolar***	***Quadripolar***
Muscle (motor) stimulation	Innervated, stimulation of motor points	Active electrode over motor point, inactive over bony prominences	×		
	Facilitation of muscle contraction for conditions like Quadriceps inhibition and deltoid inhibition	Inactive electrode over muscle origin and active over the muscle bulk		×	
	Denervated	One lead per muscle with both electrodes on the same muscle, two leads if it is a larger muscle or if the device has more than one head		×	
Sensory stimulation	Large painful area	Two leads depending on the size of the area; use as many electrodes as possible to sensory stimulation			×
	Small painful area	One lead if only one lead and two electrodes fit in the treatment area		×	
	Spinal nerve root placement	One lead with one electrode at the spinal nerve root and the other in the sensory area	×		
Relief through delivery of medication to tissues		One lead and one electrode in the treatment area and the other more proximally placed on soft tissue	×		
Wound healing	On the wound to heal it (in different stages)	One electrode in the wound and other one to complete the circuit	×		
	On the side of the wound to increase blood supply	Electrodes are placed on either side of the wound		×	
Relief of edema	Faradism under pressure	If possible two leads. Stimulating two electrodes at one time		×	
	Small area	One electrode at edematous site	×		

31

Current Flow in the Tissue

Figure 31.1 shows an electrical model for two electrodes placed on the skin surface. Skin under the electrode act as insulator whereas tissue beneath skin is conductor. So, this model where two conductors are separated by insulator or capacitor. Skin is a partial insulator because it has conductive channels created by skin appendages. C is the capacitance of stratum corneum and r is in parallel with C, represents conductive pathway by skin appendages.

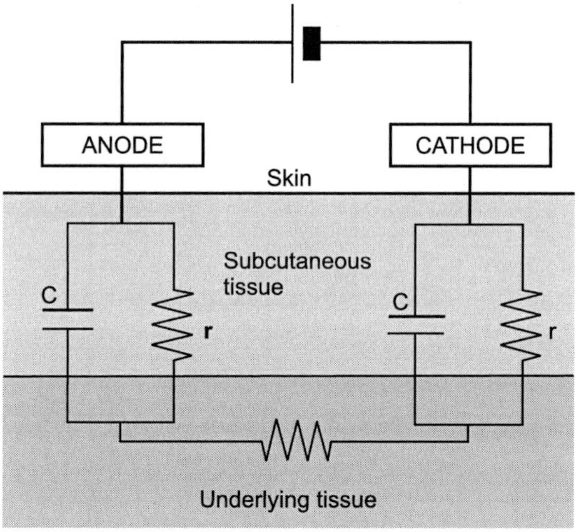

Fig. 31.1: Electrical model under the electrodes

CURRENT FLOW THROUGH SKIN

Response for a Steady Direct Current

When a steady direct current flows, initially it goes through capacitor than resister. As the capacitors are uncharged it will not offer any resistance to the current flow. As the capacitor charges, the potential difference across the capacitor increases and this opposes further flow of current. When it is fully charged the capacitor has infinite resistance, the current flow will be lower as there is current flow only through resistors. As the skin resistance is high, the potential difference across the skin is small. So nerve fibers are insensitive to steady state direct current and they are not used for stimulation of nerve fiber. The second reason why nerves are relatively insensitive to steady DC is they accommodate. That's why steady state current is used for the iontophoresis because without nerve stimulation chemicals to be driven is charged.

Response to a Pulsed Direct Current

If a pulsed direct current is applied, the initial current flow through tissue is large but it quickly drops as the capacitors charge. The time constant for charging process is proportional to R and C.

If a long pulse duration is used, the capacitors charge during the pulse and the current quickly drops to resistive current flow only. This means that if skin resistance is more, the current will drop to a very low value. At the end of the applied voltage pulse the capacitors discharge, producing a negative going current spike. So, the resulting current is effective at starting and at the end of applied voltage pulse. Most of the applied voltage is ineffective.

If the short pulse duration is used, the current decreases only fractionally during the pulse and most of the resulting current is due to the capacitors charging. The resulting current through tissue is high and does not decrease much during the pulse. The pulse duration is too short compared to time constant ($R \times C$). Most of the applied voltage is effective.

Electrical Stimulation of Nerve Fiber

Electrical stimulation of the nerve fiber involves current flow across the membrane and through intracellular fluid. So, the nerve membrane is made up of capacitance (insulating phospholipid layer) and resistance (conductive channels in the membrane). Since the membrane acts as capacitor, if alternating current is used for nerve stimulation, the PD across the membrane will be less and it will be more in the tissue below membrane at higher current frequencies. So at high frequencies, nerve fibers are less excitable because the potential difference produced across the fiber membrane is reduced. ***It is not the potential difference across the fiber determines excitation of the nerve, the potential difference across the fiber membrane determines the excitability***. So, high frequency alternating currents are not effective for nerve stimulation.

Hot Spot

Q. 1. Why steady state direct current cannot be used to for NEMS?

Ans: Nerve fibers are located deep to the skin. Most of the applied voltage drop happens at stratum corneum itself. So, the stimulation intensity reaching the nerve fiber is too low. Another reason is accommodation. The firing threshold progressively increases with a constantly applied DC stimulus. So, the nerve fiber will cease firing once the threshold has risen above the applied DC stimulus.

Q. 2. Why short duration pulse is less painful compared to long duration pulse?

Ans: A long duration pulse is effective only at the beginning and the end of a pulse. As the duration is more than the time constant, most of the applied voltage is ineffective in the deeper tissue where motor nerve is present. Most of the applied voltage dissipates in the skin where the sensory nerves (pain) are present.

Contd.

A short duration pulse shorter than the time constant so most of the applied voltage is effective. So, the maximum effect is in the deeper tissue. A second reason is better discrimination of sensory, pain and motor nerve fiber stimulation is achieved with short duration pulses.

Q. 3. Why alternating currents are not useful for nerve stimulation?

Ans: At high frequencies, nerve fibers are less excitable because the potential difference produced across the fiber membrane is reduced. It is not the potential difference across the **fiber** determines excitation of the nerve, the potential difference across the **fiber membrane** determines the excitability of the nerve. So, high frequency alternating currents are not effective for nerve stimulation.

Q. 4. Why short duration pulses intensity has to be increased?

Ans: With a very short duration pulse there is insufficient time for the membrane capacitance to fully charge and change in membrane potential is small. So, to compensate this intensity has to be increased.

Q. 5. Why denervated muscles are sensitive to long duration pulses?

Ans: The lack of neural input causes increased sensitivity of the muscle fiber membrane. The increase may be the result of normal control mechanisms whereby muscle fiber adapts to or compensates for changes in neural activity.

Q. 6. Why large diameter fibers requires less current to activate compared to small diameter fibers with electrical stimulation?

Ans: As the diameter increases, the distance between two adjacent nodes of ranvier increases. The initiation of action potential relies on producing a potential difference between adjacent nodes. Greater the intermodal distance greater will be the potential difference between two adjacent nodes for a given stimulus intensity. The larger diameter membrane has more ion channels in an average cell. This reduces resistance of the membranes. This lowers input current needed to depolarize threshold voltage. This could be another reason for recruitment.

Q. 7. Why larger fibers are recruited and fired compared to smaller fibers?

Ans: Smaller diameter fibers refractory period is longer as compared to larger diameter fibers so, their firing rates are typically less as compared to larger fibers.

Q. 8. What are the characteristics of an electrical impulse that influence its ability to stimulate nerve fibers?

Ans: There are three characteristics, they are:

- Size or amplitude of the pulse: more the amplitude more rapidly the nerve fiber will reach threshold.
- Width of duration of the pulse: longer the pulse duration, more time is available for the fiber to reach threshold.
- Rate of change or rise of the pulse: A stimulus pulse which rises slowly to its maximum value is less effective than a sudden sharp pulse. If a slow rising pulse is used then the minimum amplitude needed to elicit an action potential will be greater.

Q. 9. Will electrical stimulation evoke a motor response in a muscle where nerve supply is intact, by a direct effect on the *muscle fibers* or indirectly via excitation of *motor nerve fibers*? If so, why?

Ans: By Nerve fibers. Many muscles are deeply located and so less likely to be stimulated than those closer to the stimulating electrodes. Another reason is that the time constant for depolarization of muscle fiber is much greater than that of a nerve fiber. If short duration pulses are used, muscle fibers do not have sufficient time to respond. Nerve fibers have smaller time constant and depolarize more rapidly, are more likely to have sufficient time to reach threshold and fire.

Q. 10. Why Rectangular pulses are preferred for a normally innervated muscle?

Ans: The short rise time of a rectangular pulse overcomes the problem of accommodation of the nerve fiber membrane. There is less sensory stimulation with short duration pulse. With a long duration pulse more current is lost in the skin and subcutaneous areas where they stimulate sensory nerves. This is unpleasant and painful as compared to short duration pulses.

Q. 11. Why it is not impossible to elicit a motor response without also electrically activating sensory fibers?

Ans: The range of diameter of sensory fibers overlaps with that of motor neurons. This results in simultaneous elicitation of nerve fibers. Sensory nerve fibers are more superficial and motor nerve fibers are deep. Hence, sensory nerve fibers are closer to electrodes. This also will produce sensory stimulation.

Q. 12. Why faradic currents stimulate nerves and galvanic currents stimulate muscles?

Ans: The time constant for depolarization of a muscle fiber is much greater than that of a nerve fiber. Faradic currents are short duration pulses, duration less than the time constant for muscle fibers, nerve fibers have smaller time constant depolarizes more rapidly and are more likely to have sufficient time to reach threshold and fire.

Q. 13. What is "Time constant"? Why is it important?

Ans: Time constant is the time for capacitor to charge and discharge through resistor. If the time constant is more than the pulse duration of electrical stimulation, the intesity has to be increased to produce a contraction.

32

Stimulation of Healthy Muscle, Denervated Muscle and Stimulation for Tissue Repair

STIMULATION OF INNERVATED (HEALTHY) MUSCLE

The innervated muscle can be stimulated by Faradic currents (FC) and galvanic currents (GC). FC produces tetanic contraction so surging is used to ensure relaxation. GC produces brisk contraction. When stimulation is applied to the nerve trunk all the muscle supplied by the nerve gets stimulated. When a current is applied direct over the innervated muscle it stimulates motor point. If a longer duration current is used to stimulate, it cannot discriminate between nerve fibers so it'll be painful for the patient. If a short duration current is used, it can discriminate the different nerve fibers so it is not painful for the patient. If a long duration current is used less intensity is required to stimulate a muscle whereas if a short duration current is used more intensity is required to stimulate a muscle. For each reduction in long duration current same intensity of current is required to produce contractions. For each reduction of short duration current the intensity has to be increased. The strength of contraction depends on number of motor unit activate which further depends on intensity. Nerve has a property of accommodation. Hence, the current that rises or fall suddenly is used. Muscle contraction can be produced during the break and make of the circuit (make means circuit is on or closed; break means circuit is off or open). When the circuit is on, area under the cathode action potential is produced and it is called Cathode Closing Contraction (CCC). When the circuit is on, area adjacent to the anode action potential is produced and it is called Anode Closing Contraction (ACC). When the circuit is off area under the anode, there is sudden loss of positive charge. This can produce action potential which is called Anode Opening Contraction (AOC). When the circuit is off area adjacent to the cathode, action potential is produced which is called as Cathode Opening Contraction (COC).

Hence, CCC > ACC > AOC > COC.

The nerve has the property of accommodation. In order to prevent accommodation fast rising pulse is used (Rectangular). So, in this case cathode is used as an active electrode for innervated muscle.

STIMULATION OF DENERVATED MUSCLE

Denervated muscle can only be stimulated by galvanic current (GC). FC are not tolerated by the patient. GC produces sluggish/worm like contraction in denervated muscle. GC stimulates the muscle directly rather than motor point. If sensory nerve is not intact, Patient will not get sensation so they won't feel pain. This can result in burn due to more delivery of current. If the sensory nerve is intact, patient feel burning or stabbing sensation. More the denervation, more the longer duration current is used. For each reduction in long duration current intensity has to be increased. For short duration currents denervated muscle will not respond. Strength of contraction depends on the number of muscle fiber under the electrode which again depend on intensity. Muscle doesn't have the property of accommodation so slow rising pulse is used. If a fast rising current is used, it produces unwanted stimulation of nearby muscle and sensory stimulation which results in burns. When stimulating a denervated muscle either cathode or anode can be used as active electrode.

STIMULATION FOR TISSUE REPAIR

Tissue healing may be promoted directly by applying the current to a wound or may be promoted indirectly by controlling edema or promoting transdermal delivery of medications. The microcurrents, direct current and HVPGS are commonly used for tissue healing. These current induces Galvanotaxis, inhibition of bacterial growth and repolarises depolarised membrane.

1. **Galvanotaxis:** The word 'Galvano' means a cell producing direct current and the word 'taxis' means the orderly arrangement of motile organisms in response to a stimulus. This is referred as attraction or repulsion of cells towards injured site.

   Specific cells including neutrophils, macrophages, lymphocytes and fibroblast can be attracted to an injured healing area by an electric charge because cells themselves carry a charge.

   Inflammatory phase

   Negatively charged cells, such as macrophages and neutrophils (inactivated) will migrate toward the anode thus, promoting the inflammatory phase (phagocytosis and autolysis) of wound healing. Thus, anode is the option of choice for the management of inflamed wounds. But activated neutrophils in case of infection are attracted towards cathode. Lymphocytes and platelets are attracted towards cathode.

   Proliferative phase

   Positively charged cell, such as fibroblasts will migrate towards cathode thus, promoting the proliferative (collagen formation) phase of wound healing. With fibroblast activation there will be increased synthesis of DNA collagen. Electric current triggers Ca channels in fibroblast cell membranes to open. There will be sudden influx of Ca which induces insulin to bind receptors. This stimulates activity of fibroblast which results in synthesis of collagen. Thus, cathode is the option of choice for the management of wounds in their proliferative phase.

   Remodeling/Maturation phase

   Positively charged cells, such as keratinocytes and epidermal cells will migrate towards the cathode thus, promoting maturation phase. Thus, cathode is the option of choice for the management of wounds in their maturation phase. Mast cells regulate the remodelling of scar.

Increased mast cell activity is associated with hypertrophic and Keloid scar. An exposure to positive polarity leads to reduction of mast cells, softens scar and achieve better cosmetic results.

2. **Repolarizing depolarized membranes**

   When tissue is injured, thereby rupturing cell membranes which result charged ions leak out of the cells. Finally wound and adjacent area becomes positively charged relative to surrounding uninjured tissue. This is called the current of injury. Electrical stimulation repolarizes this depolarized membrane and accelerates healing process.

3. **Germicidal effect:** Studies have shown that electrical currents have antimicrobial effect that destroy bacteria or by reducing bacterial growth and survival. These effects are commonly on the germs, such as Pseudomonas, straphylococcus and E. coli.

4. **Increased circulation** to injured tissues thereby accelerating the healing.

33

Faradic Current

DEFINITION

Faradic current are short duration interrupted DC of duration less than 0.1 to 10 milliseconds and frequency 50–100 Hz.

Types

1. **Original faradic:** It is an uneven alternating current first with negative phase with long duration and low intensity and then with positive phase with short duration and high intensity. This current is obtained from smart Bristow induction coil. Disadvantage is such that burns will arise due to uneven alteration of current (Fig. 33.1A).
2. **Faradic type:** It is a unidirectional direct current with short duration and high intensity. Duration is short and frequency is higher, no time for relaxation so result in Tetanic contraction (Fig. 33.1B).

(A) Original faradic **(B) Faradic type**

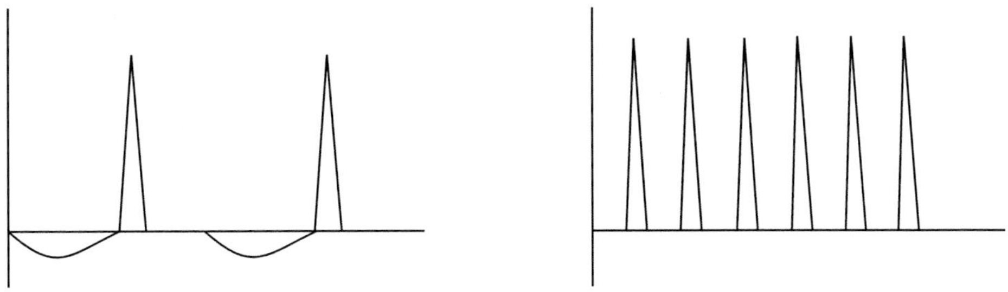

Fig. 33.1: Original faradic and faradic type currents

Synonyms: Plain faradic current or unmodified faradic current.

Difference between unmodified and modified faradic current is shown in Figure 33.2.

3. **Modified faradic current:** Intensity increases gradually. Modification is done with the help of surge.

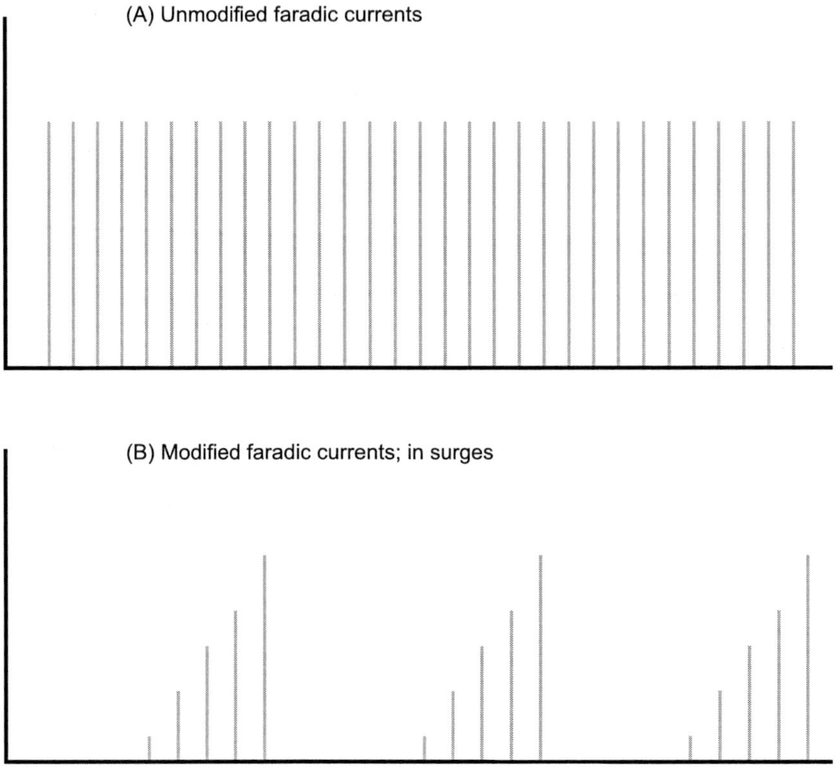

Fig. 33.2: Modified and unmodified faradic currents

SURGE

Definition: Intensity of successive impulses increases gradually. Each impulse reaching a peak value greater than the preceding one then falls either suddenly or gradually.

Purpose of surge: To produce near normal Tetanic contraction and ensure relaxation of muscles.

Performance: Surging can be done by means of hand and electronic device.

Types of Surge

- Surges varying in waveform (Fig. 33.3)
  - Saw tooth
  - Triangular
  - Trapezoid
- Surges varying in duration (Fig. 33.4)
- Varying interval between the surges (frequency) (Fig. 33.5).

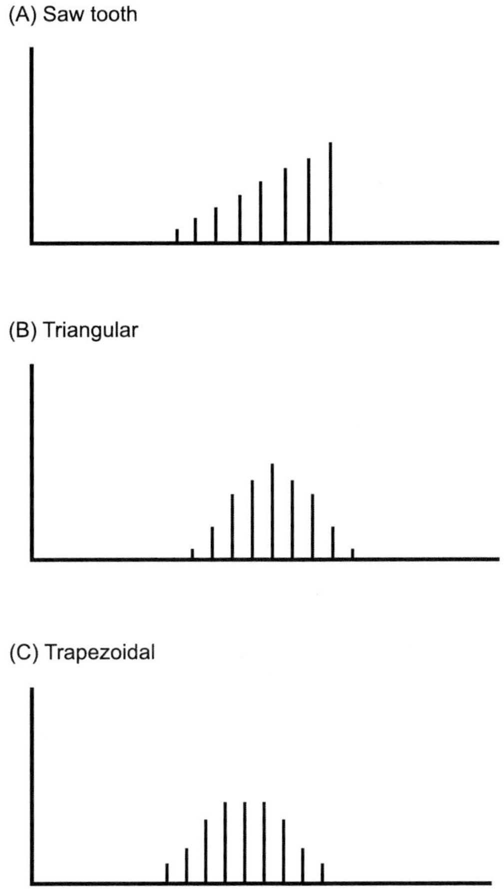

Fig. 33.3: Surges varying in waveform

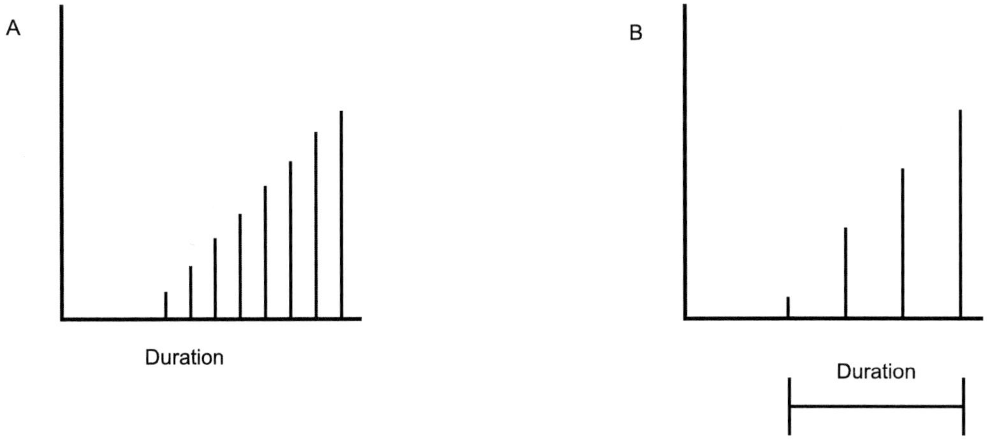

Fig. 33.4: Surges varying in duration

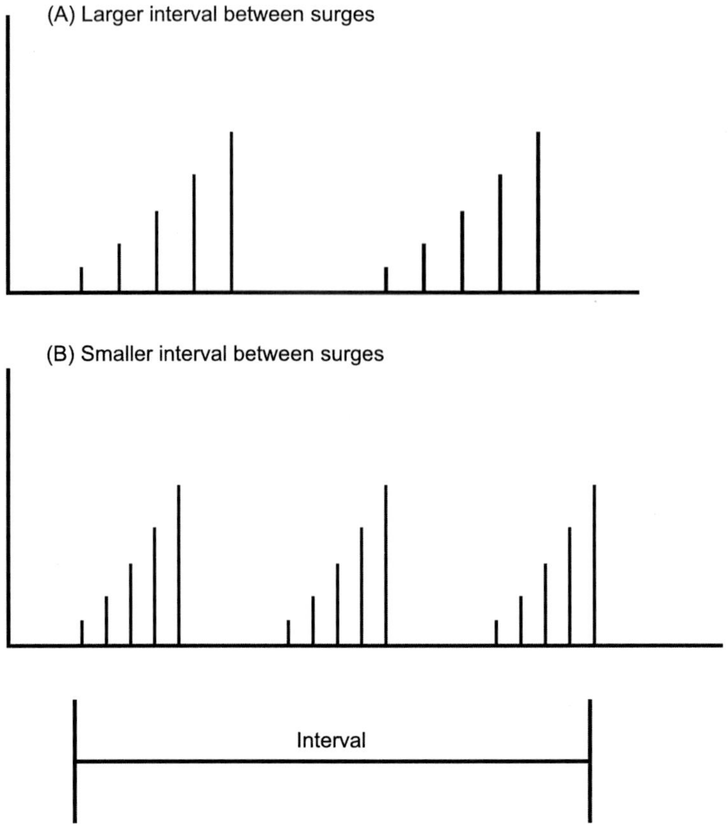

Fig. 33.5: Varying interval between surges

PHYSIOLOGICAL EFFECTS OF FARADIC CURRENT

The way the faradic current and galvanic current act on human body is almost similar so both of them is described together in Table 33.1.

Table 33.1: Physiological effect of faradic and galvanic current

Effects	*Faradic*	*Galvanic*
On sensory nerve	Pin prickling sensation	Stabbing or burning sensation
	Erythema formation (reddening of skin due to reflex vasodilation of superficial blood vessels)	
	Erythema formation is less than the galvanic as pulse duration is shorter	Erythema formation is more than the faradic as pulse duration is longer
On motor nerve		
Innervated	Tetanic	Brisk contraction
Denervated	Not tolerated by the patient	Sluggish or worm like contraction

Contd.

Contd.

Chemical effect	Less chance of chemical burn	More chance of chemical burn
	Order of chemical burn Sinusoidal > Faradic > Galvanic > Direct current	
Increase metabolism (Fig. 33.6)	More effect	Less effect
Reduction of swelling (Fig. 33.7)	More effect	Less effect

Stimulation of muscle

↓

Increased metabolism

↓

Increased demand for O_2 and nutrients

↓

Increased output of waste products (lactic acid)

↓

Dilation of arterioles and capillaries

↓

Increased blood supply to the muscle

Fig. 33.6: Increase metabolism by stimulation

Electrical stimulation

↓

Muscle contract and relax

↓

Pumping action on veins and lymphatic vessels lying within and around them

↓

Increased venous and lymphatic return

↓

Reduction of swelling

Fig. 33.7: Reduction of swelling by stimulation

Therapeutic Effects of Faradic Current

1. **Facilitation of muscle contraction:** Electrical stimulation is useful in assisting voluntary muscle contraction when a patient is unable to do muscle contraction or finds difficult to do so due to pain (As in cases of meniscotomy and ACL reconstruction).

   Suggested mechanism

   Facilitation of muscle contraction is explained as a Flowchart in the Figure 33.8 and with help of muscle spindle in the Figure 33.9.

Excitation of small efferent fibers i.e., Aγ

↓

Contraction of intrafusal muscle fiber (muscle protein contracts)

↓

Stimulation of primary nerve ending

↓

Impulse are taken by primary I a afferent to the dorsal horn

↓

Send information to large anterior horn cell

↓

Impulses are taken through Aα motor neurone

↓

Contraction of extrafusal muscle fibers

↓

At the same time inhibition of anterior horn cell supplying the antagonist

Fig. 33.8: Mechanism of facilitation of muscle contraction

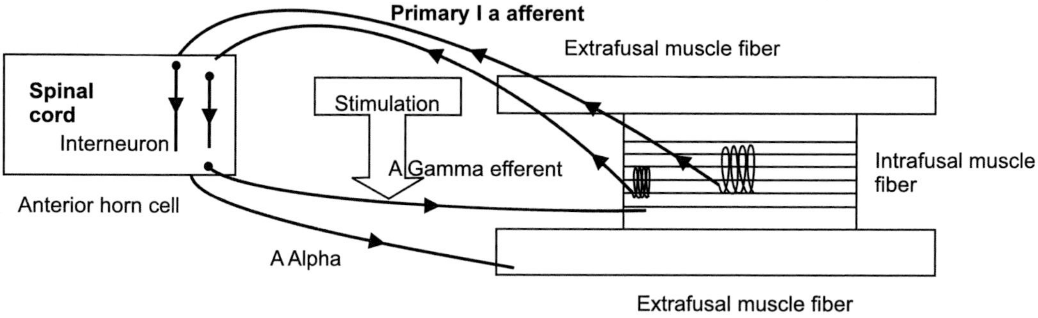

Fig. 33.9: Muscle spindle

Pain has a inhibitory effects on anterior horn cell so, it inhibits the transmission of impulse to the motor unit. On application of electrical stimulation, it reduces the inhibition on anterior horn cell thereby facilitating the muscle contraction and inducing the relaxation of antagonist muscle.

2. **Re-education of muscle action:** Inability to contract a muscle voluntarily may be due to the result of prolonged disuse in intrinsic muscle of the foot or due to incorrect use hallux valgus (due to incorrect use of abductor hallucis). Faradic stimulation is used to produce muscle contraction and helps to restore sense of movement. Brain appreciates the movement not the muscle action. Active contraction should be attempted at the same time along with electrical nerve stimulation
3. **To train a new muscle action:** In case of tendon transfer or other reconstructive surgeries, a muscle is required to perform a different action from that of the previous one. The muscle is stimulated with faradic current so its new action is performed. Patient must concentrate on the movement and attempt to assist with voluntary contraction.
4. **Neuropraxia:** In this case impulses from the brain are unable to pass the site of the lesion to reach the muscle separated by the affected nerve. So, voluntary power is reduced or lost which results in

muscle wasting. There is no degeneration of nerve in case of Neuropraxia so that if it is stimulated with faradism below the site of the lesion, the impulses pass to the muscle causing them to contract.

For example: In case of carpal tunnel syndrome, Saturday night palsy etc.

5. **Severe motor nerve:** When a nerve has been severed the degeneration of axon takes place so the faradic currents are given during earlier part of degeneration and the later part of regeneration.
6. **Improve venous and lymphatic drainage:** Faradic current contraction mimics normal muscle contraction so, the pumping action of alternate muscle contraction and relaxation and of the joint movement results in increase venous and lymphatic return. Hence, it is used for the treatment of edema and gravitational ulcer.
7. **Prevention and loosening of adhesion:** When there is effusion into the tissue and adhesions are liable to form which can be prevented by keeping the structures moving with respect to each other. So, faradic stimulation can be given to loosen the adhesion by muscle contraction.

   For example: Scar tissue binding the muscles or tendon.
8. **Counter-irritation:** The faradic current may be used to relieve pain by counter irritation. If a strong faradic current is applied in the region of sensory nerve which conducts pain transmission, the nerve adaptation takes place and its conductivity is reduced. When the stimulation ceases the nerve returns to its previous condition but it is found that the excitability is reduced and some relief of pain is obtained.

INDICATIONS OF FARADIC CURRENT

- **Facilitation of muscle contraction**
  - ACL reconstruction
  - Meniscotomy
  - Rotation cuff repair
  - Arthroscopy surgery of shoulder
  - Achilles' tendon repair
- **Re-education of muscle action**
  - Hallux valgus
  - Flat feet
  - Metatarsalgia
  - Incontinence due to pelvic floor muscle weakness
  - Incontinence after prostate surgery
  - Utero-vaginal prolapse
- **Training a new muscle action**
  - Tendon transfer
  - Muscle transfer
  - Nerve graft

  - Hysterical paralysis
  - Cerebral palsy
- **Neuropraxia**
  - Carpal tunnel syndrome
  - Saturday night palsy
  - Cubital tunnel syndrome
  - Tardy nerve palsy
  - Sciatica
  - Tarsal tunnel syndrome
- **Severed motor nerve**
  - Axillary nerve injury due to fracture of surgical neck of humerus
  - Radial nerve injury due to fracture of shaft of humerus
  - Ulnar nerve injury due to fracture of lower end of humerus
  - Posterior interosseous injury due to fracture of head of radius
  - Wrist drop, foot drop, finger drop, thumb drop
  - Fracture of head of fibula leads to deep peroneal nerve injury
  - Erbs palsy
  - Klumpkes paralysis
- **Increased venous and lymphatic return**
  - Lymphedema due to removal of breast (mastectomy)
  - Lymphedema at lower limb due to Filariasis (mosquito bite)
  - Edema due to venous disorder
  - Gravitational ulcer
  - Venous ulcer
- **Prevention and loosening of adhesion**
  - Mobilize the scar with underneath tissue stimulation
  - To mobilize the tendon
  - To mobilize the muscle from skin due to adhesion
- **Scoliosis**
- **To reduce spasticity**
- **In bell's palsy to stimulate the nerve trunk; upper, middle and lower**
- **To increase range of motion due to post traumatic stiffness**

34

Different Methods of Application of Faradic Currents

The different methods of application are as follows:

- Pelvic floor re-education
- Faradic under pressure
- Faradic foot bath
- Group muscle stimulation
- Stimulation of motor point
- Faradism under tension.

PELVIC FLOOR RE-EDUCATION

Definition

Pelvic floor muscle re-education is the faradic stimulation technique to stimulate pelvis floor muscles thereby strengthening the muscles.

Hot Spot

Since muscle of pelvic floor is thin and fatigue rapidly, the duration of treatment should therefore be short so faradic current is preferred.

Mechanism

In order to increase the bulk and power of the muscle it is necessary for it to contract on adequate number of times against the resistance of a suitable load and these conditions may be fulfilled if a muscle is to be strengthened as a result of electrical stimulation. The electrical stimulation is necessary to such active exercise as can be performed and when adequate exercise possible the later is more satisfactory method of restoring muscle power than electrical stimulation.

Indications

- Prolapse of pelvic organs like 'uterovaginal prolapse'
- Stress incontinence
- Surgical removal of prostate gland.

Equipment

- Rectal or vaginal electrode
- Rubber electrode
- Stimulator
- Wire
- Plinth.

Technique of Application (Described in Chapter 40)

- **Pre-application task**
- **Preparation of apparatus:**
  - **Testing the machine**
  - **Adjust the duration of surge and duration between the surge**
  - **Machine should be 4 m away from SWD machine.**
- **Prepare the patient psychologically**
- **Prepare the patient physically**
- **Position of the patient:** Place the patient in side lying position with pillow between lower legs. Place the plastic sheets under the patient.
- **Preparation of electrodes:**
  - Choose the appropriate electrodes
  - Put the appropriate medium of conduction
  - Fixation of electrode
  - Choosing the active and inactive electrode.
- **Placement of electrode:** The indifferent electrode with a large pad is secured on the lumbosacral region. Sterilized lubrication jelly is rubbed on the vaginal electrode which is then inserted into vagina. If no vaginal electrode is available or if this site is unstable, place a large button electrode over the urogenital region. For male patients suffering from incontinence following prostatectomy may be treated with rectal electrode.
- **Procedure:** Select a suitable duration and frequency of surge to gain a good contraction of muscle than increase the intensity gradually unit a strong contraction is achieved.

  Contraindications, dangers and precautions are same as that of faradic currents.

FARADISM UNDER PRESSURE

Definition

Electrical stimulation of muscles by using the faradic current that generally acts as the muscle pump. The compression and elevation of the limb is to increase venous and lymphatic return so relieves edema

Mechanism

Improved lymphatic and venous drainage. Pumping action of lymphatic and venous vessels by alternate contraction and relaxation of muscle and joint increases venous and lymphatic drainage (Fig. 33.7).

Principles

- Elevation by pillows: helps in Gravity assisted drainage
- Compression: by crepe bandage
- Voluntary muscle contraction
- Stimulation.

Indications

- Gravitational edema
- Lymphedema in upper limb due to removal of breast
- Lymphedema in lower limb due to Filariasis
- Venous edema/ulcers
- Post-phlebitis syndrome.

Equipment Required

- Four carbon rubber electrodes
- Pillow
- Stimulator
- Crepe bandage: 6 inch for lower limb and 4 inch for upper limb.

Technique of Application (Described in Chapter 40)

- **Pre application task**
- **Preparation of apparatus**
- **Preparation of patient psychologically**
- **Preparation of patient physically**
- **Position of patient:** Supine lying for lower limb and sitting or supine lying for upper limb
- **Preparation of electrodes**
- **Placement of electrode:** Any of the three methods can be used which is described below:
  - **First method:** Covering motor point method, Place the electrodes such a way that it covers motor points of main muscle groups that involved in the muscle pump, e.g., for lower limb one

electrode over calf muscle and one over plantar aspect of foot, for upper limbs place electrodes over flexor aspect of the forearm and arm.

- **Second method:** Nerve conduction method, Place the electrodes such a way that it stimulate the nerves directly which results in contraction of all muscles supplied by that nerve. Active electrode is placed over the nerve trunk where it is superficial.
- **Third method:** called as alternate method which is described below.

In upper limb

- 1st Electrode: Palmar aspects of hand
- 2nd Electrode: Lower aspect of flexor compartment of forearm
- 3rd Electrode: Lower arm (flexor side) or cubital fossa
- 4th Electrode: Upper arm (flexor side)
- 5th Electrode: Nape of the neck (Optional).

In lower limb

- 1st Electrode: Sole of foot
- 2nd Electrode: Calf muscle
- 3rd Electrode: On popliteal fossa
- 4th Electrode: Posterior compartment of thigh
- 5th Electrode: Lumbosacral region (Optional).

After placing electrodes apply crepe bandage starting distally. It should be firm but not too tight.

Treatment Sequence

Treatment is alternated between any two adjacent electrodes starting from distally.

- 1st session: First and second electrode, 1st cathode and 2nd anode
- 2nd session: Second and third electrode, 2nd cathode and 3rd anode
- 3rd session: Third and fourth electrode, 3rd cathode and 4th anode
- 4th session: Fourth and fifth (or first) electrode, 4th cathode and 5th or 1st anode.

Procedure: The rate of contraction must be slow, to allow maximum contraction of the muscles. The repetition rate must be slow to give time for relaxation and to allow the vessels time to refill. The typical timing for each session should be 2 to 3 minutes contraction followed by rest of 5 minutes. The total treatment time should not exceed 35 minutes.

Contraindications, dangers and precautions are same as that of faradic currents.

FARADIC FOOT BATH

Definition

The electrical stimulation of the muscles by using the faradic type current to stimulate thereby contracting intrinsic muscle of foot which further prevents the hallux valgus, foot flat, metatarsalgia putting the leg in bath is called faradic foot bath.

Mechanism

The therapeutic effect of faradic current used here is re-education of muscle action. Inability of muscle contract voluntarily may be the result of prolonged disuse or incorrect use. Faradic stimulation is used to produce the contraction and help to restore the sense of movement. Active contraction should be attempted at the same time along the electrical nerve stimulation.

Indications

- Flat feet
- Hallux valgus
- Meta tarsalgia
- Plantar fasciitis
- Calcaneal spur
- Rheumatoid arthritis of food.

Equipment Required

- Carbon rubber electrode
- Tray with saline tap water
- Pen electrode
- Wooden foot stool
- Therapeutic electric stimulator.

Technique of Application

- **Pre-application task**
- **Preparation of apparatus**
- **Preparation of patient psychologically**
- **Preparation of patient physically**
- **Position of the patient:** Sitting in a chair, back well supported. Place the patients foot in a bath containing enough warm water to cover the toes.
- **Preparation of electrode**
- **Placement of electrodes:** Described below:

  For lumbrical

  - Two electrodes placement, transversely across the bottom of the bath
  - Inactive electrode: under the heel
  - Active electrode: under the first metatarsal head.

  For planter interossei

  - On each side of foot at shaft of 1st and 5th metatarsal of shaft/head.

Abductor hallucis longus

- Place inactive electrode under the heel
- Active electrode will be a pen electrode placed on the motor point of abductor hallucis muscle.

Procedure: Select a suitable duration and frequency of surge to gain a good contraction followed by complete relaxation of the muscle. Produce several gentle contractions to allow the patient to become accustomed to the current. Then increase the intensity gradually until a strong contraction is achieved. Encourage the patients to contract the muscles voluntarily with the current. Once the patients achieve a good muscle contraction, discontinue the electrical stimulation.

Contraindications, dangers and precautions are same as that of faradic currents.

GROUP MUSCLE STIMULATION (FOR DELTOID AND QUADRICEPS INHIBITION)

Introduction

When a group of muscle is subjected for the stimulation, the faradic types of current are used. This is used when the muscles are inhibited due to pain (commonly quadriceps and deltoid).

Mechanism

Stimulation of the muscle results in facilitation of muscle contraction (mechanism explained in Figures 33.8 and 33.9) which helps in performing normal action of the muscle thereby performing normal action of the muscle which they are subjected to do so.

Indications

Indication of deltoid inhibition:

- Fracture of shaft of humerus
- Traumatic synovitis
- Any soft tissue injury around the shoulder joint
- Dislocation of shoulder joint
- Fracture of surgical perk of humerus
- All arthroscopic rotator cuff.

Indications of quadriceps inhibition:

- Fracture of shaft of femur
- Meniscotomy
- Traumatic synovitis of knee
- Surgical intervention
- Soft tissue injury around the knee.

Equipment Required

- Carbon rubber electrode: size (12 * 9 cm) and (15 * 8 cm)
- Therapeutic electric stimulator
- Straps
- Jaconet
- Arm sling or modified towel
- Pillow.

Technique of Application (Described in Chapter 40)

- **Pre-application task**
- **Preparation of apparatus**
- **Preparation of patient psychologically**
- **Preparation of patient physically**
- **Position of the patient**
  - **For quadriceps inhibition:** Long sitting position with back supported, with 15 degree of flexion (pillow under knee).
  - **For deltoid inhibition:** Sitting in a chair without side rest with affected limb in a arm sling so that arm can freely move with stimulation and voluntary contraction.
- **Preparation of electrode**
- **Placement of electrodes: Described below.**

  For Quadriceps inhibition
  - Inactive electrode: Upper 1/3th of thigh (femoral triangle)
  - Active electrode: Over the lower part of thigh.

  For deltoid inhibition
  - Inactive electrode: Origin of the deltoid muscle near acromion process
  - Active electrode: Over anterior and middle fibers of deltoid.
- **Procedure:** Select a suitable duration and frequency of surge to gain a good contraction followed by complete relaxation of the muscle. Produce several gentle contractions to allow the patient to become accustomed to the current. Then increase the intensity gradually until a strong contraction is achieved. Encourage the patients to contract the muscles voluntarily with the current. Once the patients achieve a good muscle contraction, discontinue the electrical stimulation.

  Contraindications, dangers and precautions are same as that of faradic currents.

STIMULATION OF MOTOR POINTS

This method has the advantage that each muscle performs its own individual action and that the optimum contraction of each can be obtained. This method is generally used to train a new action for the muscle or a specific muscle is weak, e.g., VMO. The inactive electrode is placed in a far area especially on a bony prominence. Active electrode is placed over a motor point. In a superficially placed muscle the motor point is at the junction of upper and middle one third where it is fleshy. For deeply placed muscles satisfactory stimulations can be obtained when it is stimulated where they emerge superficially.

FARADISM UNDER TENSION

This method is commonly used in physiotherapy management following plastic surgeries especially after tendon sutures or scar tissue binding muscle and tendon or fascia. After these surgeries adhesions are liable to form which can be prevented by keeping the structures moving with respect to each other by stimulation. So faradic currents can prevent or loosen these adhesions. For the method of stimulation, the inactive electrode is placed over the convenient area and active electrode is placed over muscle belly of tendon repaired. If the motor points are inaccessible because of wound or splinting, active electrode can be placed over the nerve trunk where it becomes superficial.

35

Galvanic Current

DEFINITION

Galvanic current are long duration interrupted direct current of duration more than 10 milliseconds and of frequency 30 Hertz.

Types

It can be any of the following:

- Fast rising current
  (a) Rectangular
- Slow rising current
  (a) Saw tooth
  (b) Triangular
  (c) Trapezoid
- Depolarized pulse

Hot Spot

Preference of fast rising current versus slow rising current on muscle stimulation.

Muscle	*Fast rising current*	*Slow rising current*
Innervated	✓ Nerve has the property of accommodation so if Fast rising current is used, it never adapts or accommodates.	× Not used. Because nerve has the property of accommodation so, greater current is required for subsequent contraction.

Contd.

Contd.

Denervated	× Produces unwanted stimulation of nearby muscle so, more current is required. Also produces more sensory stimulation so, patient will not allow.	✓ You can eliminate unwanted stimulation of nearby muscle. So, less current is required to produce muscle contraction.

More the muscle is denervated, more the slow rising pulse is preferred, e.g., Trapezoidal.

More the muscle is denervated, long duration is used, e.g., 300 ms.

More the muscle is re-innervated, shorter duration is used like 0.01ms. The duration between the pulses or pulse interval should be more than that of pulse duration.

Depolarized pulse: To reduce chemical burn, the current is given in opposite direction.

PHYSIOLOGICAL EFFECT OF GALVANIC CURRENTS

Comparison with faradic currents is detailed in Table 33.1.

- On sensory nerve:
  - Burning or stabbing sensation
  - Erythema formation due reflex vasodilation of superficial blood vessels as current remains longer.
- On motor nerve:
  - Innervated: Brisk contraction
  - Denervated: Sluggish or worm like contraction.
- Chemical effect:
  - More chance of chemical burn
  - When a current passes through electrode chemical changes takes place at the tissue, i.e., opposite charge particle accumulates under the electrode which results in electrolysis which in turn results in chemical burn.
  - More burns happen with longer duration, e.g., 300–1000 ms.
- On metabolism and venous and lymphatic circulation (Figs. 33.6 and 33.7).
  - Less effect is seen compared to FC.

THERAPEUTIC EFFECTS

In case of severe motor nerve galvanic currents are given in the later part of degeneration and earlier stage of regeneration. In case of later part of degeneration start with 10 ms of duration, if not responding progress to the next longer duration and finally up to 1000 ms. In case of earlier part of re-innervation start with 1000 ms of duration and go to short duration and finally up to 10 ms. Once the good response is achieved with shorter duration, switch back to faradic current (Table 35.1).

Table 35.1: Nerve injury stages and current administered

Stage	***Days***	***Current administered***	***Phase***
Nerve injury ↓ Starting of Wallerian degeneration	Day 0 | Day 14	Faradic	Faradic currents at the early stages of denervation
↓	|	Faradic Galvanic 10 30	Galvanic currents at the late stages of denervation
Degeneration complete Regeneration starts	Day 28 |	100 300 1000 1000	Galvanic currents at the early stages of renervation
↓ Regeneration completed	Regeneration at @ 1 mm/day	300 100 30 10 Faradic	Faradic currents at the late stages of renervation

Rationale of Administering Galvanic Currents to a Denervated Muscle

Why electric stimulation has to be given in a denervated muscle is detailed in Figure 35.1.

When a nerve to a muscle is cut
↓
Muscle paralysis
↓
Muscle wasting
↓
Muscle fibrosis
↓
Properties of muscles are lost

Fig. 35.1: Rationale of muscle stimulation for a denervated muscle

Property of Muscle

Extensibility: Muscle can be stretched.

Elasticity: If we release the stretch, muscle comes back to normal length.

Irritability: Once the nerve is stimulated muscle is excited.

Contractility: Once it is excited, the muscle is contracted.

Electrical Stimulation Maintains the Property of Muscle Till the Reinnervation Happens

Indications:

- Fracture of surgical neck of humerus.
- Fracture of shaft of humerus causes radial nerve palsy results in paralysis of wrist extensor, which results in wrist drop, finger drop.
- Fracture of lower end of humerus result in the ulnar nerve palsy results in paralysis of hypothenar muscle and flexor carpi ulnaris, ADM, AP results in Claw hand.
- Fracture of head of the radius results in injury to posterior interosseous nerve results in Paralysis of deep extensor (ECRL, ECRB, BR) results in Finger drop, Wrist drop.
- Brachial plexus injury:
  - Erb's palsy
  - Klumpke's palsy.
- Carpal tunnel syndrome with severe compression.
- Injury to sciatic nerve like in case of foot drop.
- Fracture of head of fibula results in injury to peroneal nerve Foot drop.
- LMN facial palsy or bell's palsy.

Hot Spot

> The current waveform should have a pulse duration equal to or greater than the chronaxie of the denervated muscle.

36

Methods of Application of Galvanic Current

The main therapeutic use of galvanic currents is the direct stimulation of nerve fibers; therefore the treatment must be arranged so that current passes through all the fibers of the muscle.

There are various methods of application:

- Stabile technique
- Labile technique
  - Labile technique with one electrode moving
  - Labile technique with two electrode moving
- Technique of application for the kid.

STABILE TECHNIQUE

Two electrodes are used, one over the origin and other over the lower end of the muscle group to be stimulated and electrodes are fixed. All muscle fibers contract equally under electrodes (Fig. 36.1A).

- **Advantage**
  - Tendon can be palpated.
  - Permits large number of contractions.
  - Can stimulate all the muscles under the electrode.
- **Disadvantage**
  - More chance of chemical burn.
  - Current will spread to nearby muscle

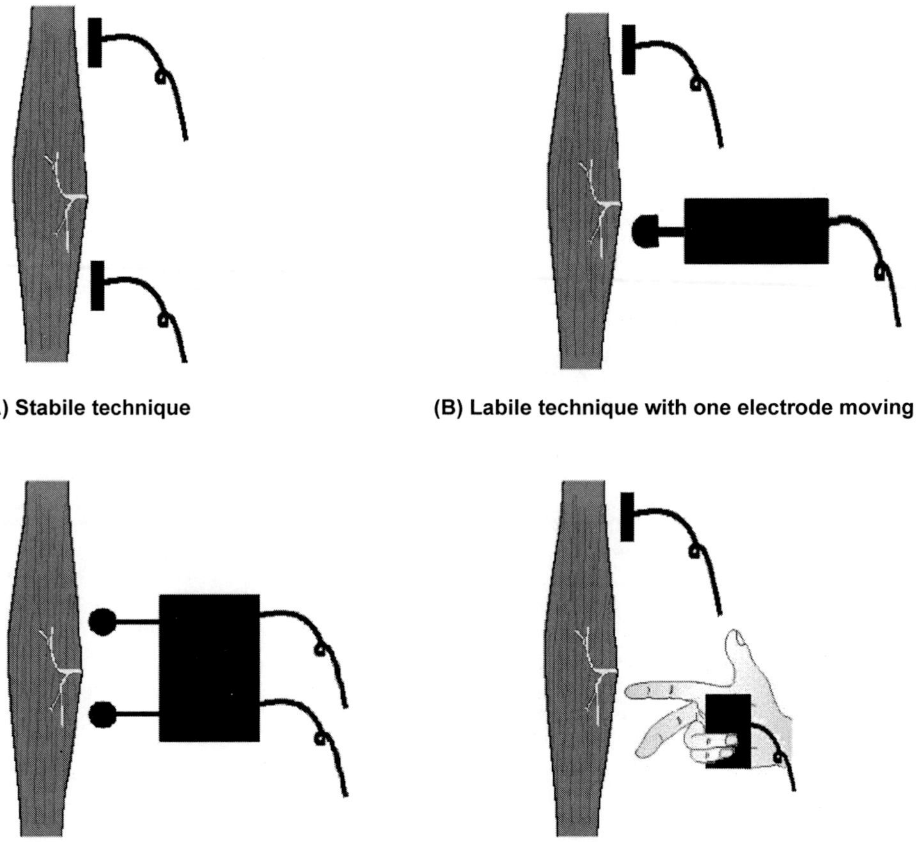
(A) Stabile technique

(B) Labile technique with one electrode moving

(C) Labile technique with both electrode moving

(D) Technique for kids

Fig. 36.1

LABILE TECHNIQUE

Labile Technique with One Electrode Moving

The inactive electrode is fixed over the bony area or origin of muscle group, the active electrode (pen electrode) will be moving in a + (plus) direction. Moving the electrode over the muscle ensures that the current passes through the maximum number of fibers (Fig. 36.1B).

- **Advantage**
  - Less chance of chemical burn.
  - Less irritation of the skin.
  - Can stimulate individual muscle.
  - When each muscle is stimulated, the other muscle in a group is rested.

- **Disadvantage**
  - Less number of muscle fibers are stimulated.
  - Cannot feel the tendon by one hand.

Labile Technique with Two Electrodes Moving

In this technique, both electrode will be moving (Fig. 36.1C).

- **Advantage**
  - It is suitable for the stimulation of deep muscle.
  - Less chance of chemical burn.
- **Disadvantage**
  - Cannot feel the tendon.
  - Difficulty in controlling the knob.
  - Tiredness to the physiotherapist.

TECHNIQUE OF APPLICATION FOR THE KID

One inactive electrode is kept in the baby's neck and active electrode is kept in therapist hand (Fig. 36.1D).

- **Advantage**
  - Less intensity of current (therapist will be able to know how much current is given).
- **Disadvantage**
  - Unwanted muscle contraction of the therapist.

37

Contraindications, Precaution and Dangers of Currents

CONTRAINDICATION

1. **Patient with cardiac pacemaker:** Electrical stimulation may interfere with pace maker and can alter the heart rate.
2. **Unstable angina (chest pain at rest):** Electrical stimulation may aggravate the rhythm disturbances due to increase work done because of stimulation.
3. **Active epiphysis region in children:** It may alter the growth of a bone.
4. **With epileptic patients:** Risk of causing an epileptic episode.
5. **Over carotid sinus:** Avoid placement of electrodes on the anterior or lateral neck because stimulation to this area may induce a rapid fall in BP and heart rate that may cause the patient to faint.
6. **Over anterior cervical area:** May stimulate vagus nerve or phrenic nerve.
7. **Venous thrombosis/arterial thrombosis:** Stimulation may increase circulation which increases the risk of releasing the thrombus (emboli).
8. **During pregnancy:** Avoid stimulation over pelvis, abdomen, trunk, lower back area where the part of the current might cross the uterus which might produce uterine contraction which results in miscarriage/abortion. Stimulation can even interfere the fetal heart rate.
9. **Malignant tumor:** Applied electrical stimulation results in increased blood supply which enhances the tissue growth and tends to spread to the other area. However, in the terminal stages of cancer IFT and TENS will be given based on physicians advice as a palliative care.
10. **Over hemorrhagic area:** Risk of enhanced bleeding due to increased blood flow in the treated area.
11. **Over osteomyelitis area:** Stimulation may produce tissue growth and may superficially cover osteomyelitis area.

12. **After radiotherapy:** After the therapy tissues may be devitalised. With stimulation tissues cannot cope up the stress produced by muscle contraction.

PRECAUTION

1. **Impaired sensation:** If there is loss of sensation in the area being treated higher intensity results in chemical burn, therefore, the intensity of the current should be administered in safe limit.
2. **Impaired mentation:** The patient with impaired mentation will be agitated and try to pull off the electrical stimulation wires so stimulation should be applied with caution and attention.
3. **Skin irritation/open wounds:** Open or damaged skin should be avoided because it has lower resistance and less sensation than the intact skin which results in too much current being delivered to the area. So, it results in chemical burn and severe pain. Some of the currents are contraindicated in open wounds.
4. **Old scar tissue:** Petroleum jelly should be applied as it prevents the current passing through the scar.
5. **Recent scar tissue/recently operated area:** If stimulation or current is given operated tissue, it will get separated.
6. **Known history of cardiac disease** like Myocardial infarction, Congenital and acquired cardiac abnormalities: Stimulation may produce some type of rhythm disturbances. Better to avoid stimulation over transthoracic area because it may alter the rhythm and may also stimulate the Intercostal muscles
7. **Electrical stimulation should not followed after any other physical agents like heat, ice, ultrasound.**
8. **Coupling media temperature in case of wound management:** Cool media may chill the wound, slows down the mitotic activity and thus, delays wound healing in HVPGS, microcurrents and DC.
9. **Those who are on with anticoagulant therapy, long-term steroid therapy:** Skin or tissue damage is likely in these patients so when applying suction electrodes care should be taken. It may result in hematoma ecchymosis due to suction force on a fragile skin.
10. **Galvanic rash:** Red or white spot or minute blister appears on the skin as a result of passage of constant direct current. The skin should be washed and smoothening cream is applied.
11. **Giddiness:** If constant direct current is passed through the TM joint or through the ear, the giddiness is liable to occur as it passes through semicircular canal. When applying the current to this area, the patient should be fully supported and current is reduced gradually.
12. **Hypertension/Hypotension:** As with stimulation it may affect the autonomic nervous system, fluctuation of blood pressure may happen. It is better to monitor BP response during treatment.

DANGERS

Burns: Patient may get electrical or chemical burn. Chemical burn arises due to application of DC and electrical burn occurs due to a shock. If there is not enough conduction medium on an electrode, as can occur with repeated use of self-adhesive electrodes or poorly applied non-adhesive electrodes the risk of burns also increases due to the increased current density. Explained in Chapter 25.

Shock: Patient may receive shock with stimulation. This may be macro shock or micro shock which is already explained in Chapter 24.

Skin irritation or inflammation: This may occur in the area where electrical stimulation electrodes are applied because the patient is allergic to the contact surface of the electrode, such as the adhesive or foam rubber. If this occurs, a different type of electrode should be tried.

Electrical stimulations may be painful: Some patients find electrical stimulation to be painful. In such patients, increasing the current amplitude slowly over a longer period of time may be better tolerated. In patients who find all forms of electrical stimulation painful, other treatment approaches should be used.

Cross infection: Infection may spread from one patient to another patient (Cross contamination) if electrodes are not sterilized and well-cleaned. It mainly happens with application of IFT and HVPGS.

Disruption of stimulating devices: Due to the proximity of diathermy equipment, which can result in altered output.

A detailed contraindications and precautions of each currents are mentioned in Table 37.1.

Table 37.1: Contraindications, precautions of electric currents

Contraindications	*Type of contra-indication*	*Macro currents*											*Micro currents*
		Low frequency DC						*Modified AC*		*Medium frequency*			
		Faradic currents	*Galvanic currents*	*Plain direct currents*	*Ionto-phoresis*	*TENS*	*HVPGS*	*Sinusoidal currents*	*Diadynamic currents*	*IFT*	*Russian*	*Rebox*	
Patient with cardiac pacemaker	General	✓	✓	✓	✓	✓	✓	✓	✓	✓	✓	✓	✓
Unstable angina (chest pain at rest)	General	✓	✓	✓	✓	✓	✓	✓	✓	✓	✓	✓	✓
Epilepsy	General	✓	✓	✓	✓	✓	✓	✓	✓	✓	✓	✓	✓
Over carotid sinus, ant cervical area	Local	✓	✓	✓	✓	✓	✓	✓	✓	✓	✓	✓	✓
Venous thrombosis/arterial thrombosis	Local	✓	✓	✓	✓	✓	✓	✓	✓	✓	✓	✓	Not known
Pregnancy	Local	✓	✓	✓	✓	✓	✓	✓	✓	✓	✓	✓	✓
Malignant tumor	Local	✓	✓	✓	✓	✓	✓	✓	✓	✓	✓	✓	✓
Hemorrhage	Local	✓	✓	✓	✓	✓	✓	✓	✓	✓	✓	✓	✓
Active epiphyseal regions in children	Local	✓	✓	✓	✓	✓	✓	✓	✓	✓	✓	✓	✓
Transcranial area	Local	✓	✓	✓	✓	✓	✓	✓	✓	✓	✓		
Infection like active tuberculosis	Local	✓	✓	✓	✓	✓	✓	✓	✓	✓	✓	✓	
Electronic implants	Local	✓	✓	✓	✓	✓	✓	✓	✓		✓	✓	
Open wounds	Local	✓	✓					✓	✓	✓	✓	✓	
Acute skin conditions: Dermatitis eczema, psoriasis, acne	Local											✓	
Osteomyelitis	Local						✓						✓
Senile or confused patients	Local									✓	✓		

Contd.

Contd.

Across the temporal and orbicular regions	Local				✓								
Known sensitivity or allergy to the therapeutic ions	Local				✓								
Precautions													
Known history of cardiac disease like Myocardial infarction		✓	✓	✓	✓	✓	✓	✓	✓	✓	✓	✓	✓
Impaired sensation		✓	✓	✓	✓	✓	✓	✓	✓	✓	✓	✓	
Impaired mentation		✓	✓	✓	✓	✓	✓	✓	✓	✓	✓	✓	
Skin irritation		✓	✓	✓	✓	✓	✓	✓	✓	✓	✓	✓	
Old scar tissue		✓	✓	✓	✓	✓	✓	✓	✓	✓	✓	✓	
Recent scar tissue/recently operated area		✓	✓	✓	✓	✓	✓	✓	✓	✓	✓	✓	
Coupling media temperature				✓	✓		✓						✓
Galvanic rash			✓	✓									
Galvanic giddiness			✓	✓									
Dangers													
Shock		✓	✓	✓	✓	✓	✓	✓	✓	✓	✓	✓	
Chemical burn		✓	✓	✓	✓	✓							
Skin irritation		✓	✓	✓	✓	✓		✓	✓	✓	✓	✓	
Painful		✓	✓	✓	✓	✓		✓	✓	✓	✓	✓	
Cross infection							✓			✓			

38

Direct Current

DEFINITION

Direct current is defined as uninterrupted direct current of unvarying intensity which is of unidirectional current.

PRODUCTION OF DIRECT CURRENT

A DC current is produced with the help of rectifier through a step down transformer (Fig. 38.1). Parts and its functions are described below:

1. Switch to on and off the circuit.
2. Step down transformer to reduce the voltage and to render the circuit earth free.

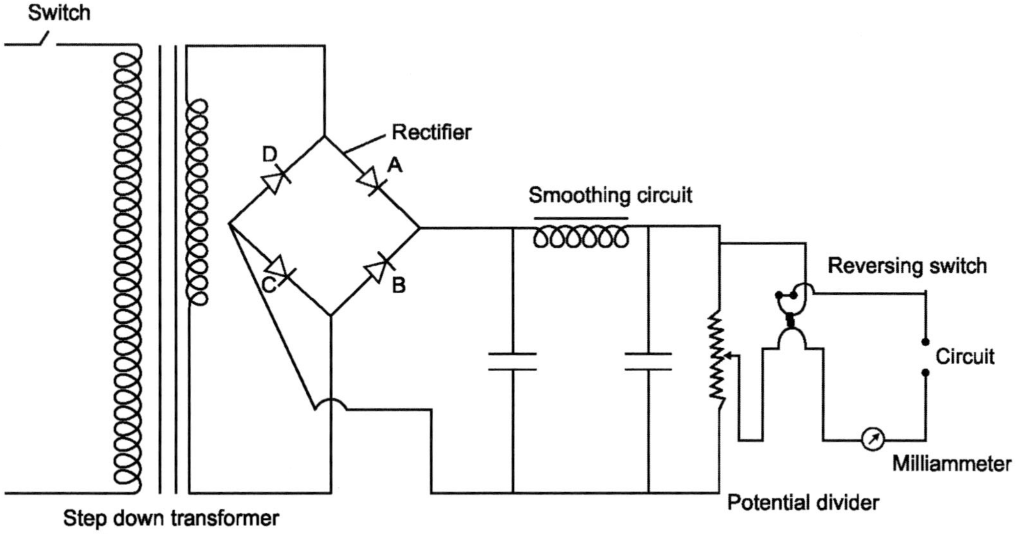

Fig. 38.1: Production of DC

3. Rectifier which converts AC to DC in full wave rectification.
4. Potential divider which varies the intensity from zero to maximum.
5. Smoothing circuit which makes the intensity rises gradually with the help of inductor (because of self induced emf) and current gradually comes to zero as the capacitor discharge slowly.
6. Reversing switch is to allow the change in direction of current.
7. Milliammeter is to show the display of current.

The construction and working of all the components are already explained in the chapters in Section A–biophysics except the reversing switch which is explained below.

REVERSING SWITCH

This device is commonly employed in DC circuit for reversing the direction of the current supplied to the patient. This can minimise chemical burns. The switch has two semicircular metal strips are joined together with the convex surfaces towards each other, but separated by insulating material. Four equidistant contacts are arranged so that one touches each end of each strip. The contacts are fixed, but the strips can be rotated through a quarter of a circle by turning a knob. Two opposite contacts, A and B are connected to the source of current, and the other two opposite contacts, C and D, to the external circuit. In Figure 38.2 A, the course of the electron flow is to A, then to C to X, then to external circuit and returned to B through D from Y, and so back to the source. In Figure 38.2 B, the strips have been rotated through a quarter of a circle. Again electrons flow to A, but this time they pass to D, to the external circuit via Y, and return via X to C, pass to B, and goes back to the source. This time the current is reversed. If a reversing switch is included in a circuit in which a one way reading milliampere meter is used, the latter must be placed before the reversing switch.

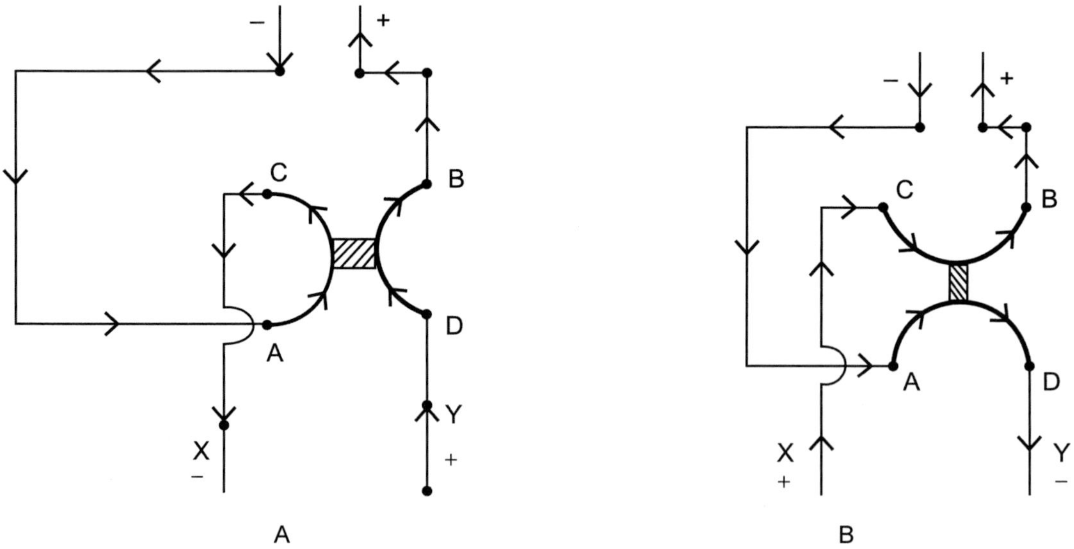

Fig. 38.2: Working of a reversing switch

PHYSIOLOGICAL EFFECTS OF DIRECT CURRENT

Two effects are seen with the application of therapeutic DC. They are interpolar effects and polar effects.

Interpolar Effect

These are produced throughout the pathway of current but most marked in superficial tissue because of higher current density. The effect seen under cathode and anode is same. The effects are mentioned below:

1. *Sensory stimulation*: Application of DC starts with tickling and prickling sensation and finally changed into irritation and itching.
2. *Hyperemia:* Erythema of skin is developed under both electrodes but more marked under anode. Erythema is confined under the area of applied electrodes. It last for 20 minutes but it may re-occur after several hours.

   #### *Causes of Erythema Due to Application of DC:*

   Moving ions stimulate sensory nerve ending which causes a reflex dilatation of blood vessel. Irritation of vessel produces liberation of H substance. This produces a triple response, i.e., dilatation, axon reflex and edema due to increased permeability. It may be by the result of mechanical action of moving ion bombarding the walls of blood vessels.
3. *Local warmth:* Increased supply of nutritive substance and elimination of waste products is accelerated which increases the further blood supply producing the warmth.

Polar Effects

These are the effects produced within the tissue under the electrode. It differs at both anode and cathode.

1. **Electrotonus:** The effects of direct current on conductivity and excitability of nerve is called as electrotonus. These effects are of two types which are mentioned below:
   (*a*) *Anelectrotonus:* There is decreased excitability and conductivity of nerve in the area under anode. Potential difference developed under the anode augment the resting potential difference and become hyperpolarized. So, it makes more difficult for an impulse to pass.
   (*b*) *Cateletrotonus:* It is the increased excitability and conductivity of nerve in the region of cathode. PD developed under the cathode reduces the resting potential difference which depolarizes the membrane and also increases conductivity of the nerve fiber.
2. **Electrophoresis:** The movement of fluid towards or away from the electrode when a current is passed through semisolid electrolyte, such as gelatine is called as electrophoresis. When DC is applied to the human body, it shows the property of electrophoresis. These effects are of two types which are mentioned below:
   (*a*) *Cataphoresis:* Increased fluid collection under the cathode by the application of DC is called as cataphoresis.
   (*b*) *Anaphoresis:* Decreased fluid collection under the anode by the application of DC is called anaphoresis.

Mechanism of electrophoresis: This is due to the movement of positively charged colloidal particle which are present in the electrolyte to which the water molecules aggregate.

3. **Relief of pain:** Both cathode and anode can be used for pain relief. Under cathode the pain relief is due to the removal of pain inducing factors due to excessive vasodilatation (Also due to counter irritation) and under the anode, pain relief is due to repulsion of hydrogen ion and K^+ ions.
4. **Chemical effect:** DC is more prone to get chemical burn then faradic and galvanic current.
5. **Introduction of ions to the tissue**: When a constant DC is passed through the body there are two way migrations of ions. Positive ions are repelled by anode and attracted by cathode. Negative ions are repelled by cathode and attracted by anode. This treatment technique as called as iontophoresis or medical ionization.
6. **Tissue damage:** At higher current density, DC will cause tissue damage. Coagulation of protein happens under anode whereas liquefaction of protein takes place under cathode. This treatment technique is also called as surgical ionization. The chemical accumulated under anode is acidic (HCl) and under cathode is alkaline. Both of this causes destruction of tissues.
7. **Acceleration of healing:** With the application of DC, there is increased chance of new bone formation and increased healing of superficial open wound by a principle called Galvanotaxis (Mechanism already explained in previous Chapter 32).

THERAPEUTIC EFFECTS

- Resolution of inflammation: because of increased blood supply to the area.
- Relief of pain due to Counter irritation, Removing the pain producing substance and Repulsion of H^+ and K^+ ions under anode.
- Softening of scar by Cataphoresis.
- Reduction of edema by Anaphoresis.
- Acceleration of healing.

METHODS OF APPLICATION

1. Iontophoresis.
2. Cathodal galvanism.
3. Anodal galvanism.
4. DC for wound healing.

INDICATIONS

- Rheumatoid arthritis.
- Osteoarthritis.
- Tenosynovitis.

- Golfer's elbow.
- Tennis elbow.
- Ankle sprain.

Contraindications, dangers and precautions are detailed in Chapter 37.

SPECIAL PRECAUTIONS OF DC

Galvanic rash: Red or white spot or minute blister appears on the skin as a result of passage of constant current. The skin should be washed and smoothening cream is applied.

Giddiness: If current is passed through the TM joint or through the ear, the giddiness is liable to occur as it passes through semicircular canal. When applying the current to this area, the patient should be fully supported and current is increased gradually.

39

Cathodal Galvanism and Anodal Galvanism

CATHODAL GALVANISM

Definition

The therapeutic effect produced under the cathode with the application of DC is called cathodal galvanism. The cathode is applied over the affected area. The circuit is completed with a larger anode elsewhere in the body.

Principle

Anode should be larger than the cathode so that the current density under anode will be less.

Duration of Treatment

20–30 minutes applied on alternate days.

PHYSIOLOGICAL EFFECTS

- Sensory stimulation
- Hyperemia
- Local warmth
- Catelectrotonus
- Cataphoresis
- *Relief of pain:* Due to removal of pain inducing factors.

- *Chemical formation:* Alkaline formation under cathode.
- *Tissue damage:* There will be liquefaction of protein.

Therapeutic Effects

- Pain relief
- Softening of scar
- To stimulate or to increase the excitability of nerve
- Post-traumatic conditions of joint like rotation cuff tendinitis.

Uses

- Resolution of chronic conditions like osteoarthritis
- Rheumatoid arthritis
- Scar tissue mobilization
- Used of lower motor neurone lesions
- Frost bite
- Post-traumatic condition of joints.

Methods of Application

A cathode pad is placed over the site of tissue. In some cases cathodal bath can be used.

ANODAL GALVANISM

Definition

The therapeutic effect produced under the anode with the application of DC is called anodal galvanism. The anode is applied over the affected area. The circuit is completed with a larger cathode elsewhere in the body.

Principle

Cathode should be larger than anode so that current density under cathode is less.

Duration

45–60 minutes can be given everyday.

Physiological Effects

- Sensory stimulation
- Hyperemia
- Local warmth
- Anelectrotonus

- Relief of pain by counter irritation
- Repulsion of H^+ and K^+ ions
- *Tissue damage:* There will be coagulation of proteins
- *Chemical accumulation:* Formation of acid (HCl) under anode.

Therapeutic Effects

- Reduces pain and muscle spasm
- Recent sports injuries
- Resolution of inflammation
- Reduction of edema.

Uses

- Ankle sprain
- Rheumatic arthritis
- Sciatica
- IV disc prolapse
- Bell's palsy
- Tenosynovitis.

Methods of Application

A large anodal pad is used to cover up swollen or painful area or an anode bath should be used.

Contraindication, Dangers, Precaution of galvanism is same as that of DC.

40

Practical Application of Electric Currents

Following are components comes under practical applications of electric currents:

- **Pre-application task**
- **Preparation of apparatus**
- **Prepare the patient psychologically**
- **Prepare the patient physically**
- **Position the patient**
- **Preparation of electrode**
- **Placement of electrodes**
- **Techniques of application.**

PRE-APPLICATION TASK

- Evaluate the injury or problem
- Look out for the contraindications
- Select the electric current characteristics
- If stimulation is applied previously review the patients response to that treatment.

PREPARATION OF APPARATUS

- Testing the machine: The operator should test the apparatus by attaching leads and electrodes to the terminals, holding the two electrodes in a moistened hand and turning up the current until expected sensation experiences or the expected muscle contraction produced. The duration of the surge and duration between the surge (rest period) should also be checked if required.
- Describe the sensation to the patient what you felt and make sure the patient can see the muscle contraction produced.
- Machine should be 4 m far from short wave diathermy.

PREPARE THE PATIENT PSYCHOLOGICALLY

- Explain the procedure
- Describe the expected sensation
- Explain about the stimulation that it produces muscle to contraction, a small amount of current will be used, it will not produce shock and it will not be painful
- Demonstrate the procedure on yourself if the patient is apprehensive.

PREPARE THE PATIENT PHYSICALLY

- Remove the clothing from electrode contact area
- Position the patient in comfortable position
- Inspect the skin for cut and abrasion
- If the area to be stimulated has hair it needs to be shaved
- Check the sensation of the skin
- Check the range of motion
- Do the methods to reduce skin resistance, washing, warming, wetting, scrapping
- A broken skin is protected by a coat of petroleum jelly.

POSITION THE PATIENT

Positioning the patient should be based on the purpose of treatment.

PREPARATION OF ELECTRODE

- Choose the appropriate electrode (rubber, metal, pen, etc.)
- Put the appropriate medium for conduction:
  - Rubber electrode: gel
  - Pen electrode: dipped in water
  - Plate electrode: lint pad with water (lint should be eight layers).
- Fixation of electrode by straps or tape or body weight or sand bag, etc.
- Choose the active and inactive electrode
- A jaconet (a kind of plastic sheeting) may be used to protect the bandage or clothing from moisture.

PLACEMENT OF ELECTRODES

Placement of electrode will be based on the purpose of stimulation and stimulator used.

TECHNIQUE OF APPLICATION

The technique will be different based on the current used and it is covered in the respective chapters.

41

Iontophoresis

HISTORY

Proposed by Le Duc in 1900.

Ionto: Ionised, *Phoresis*: Local transfer.

Definition

Transdermal application of mild direct current to drive positively charged or a negatively charged ion of a drug solution into the patient's skin and the underlying tissues.

WORKING PRINCIPLE

Like charges repel each other so that the drug ions are repelled or pushed into the skin and the surrounding tissue by direct current. The Anodal iontophoresis refers to transfer of a positively charged drug solution (Fig. 41.1) and Cathodal iontophoresis refers to transfer of a negatively charged drug solution.

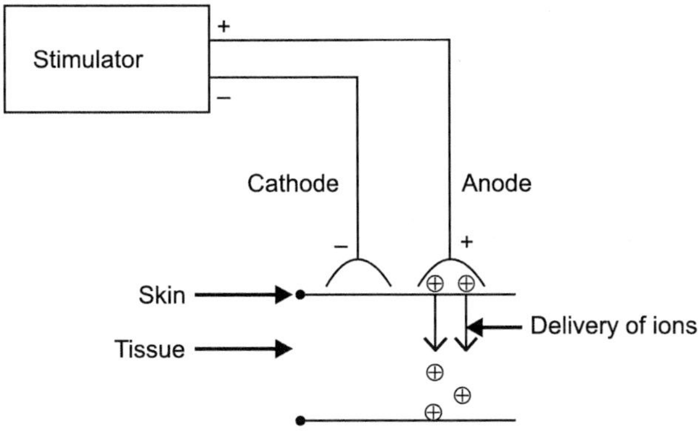

Fig. 41.1: Anodal iontophoresis

MECHANISM OF IONTOPHORESIS

Iontophoresis enhances transdermal drug delivery by various mechanisms:

Electromigration/Electrorepulsion: Ion electric field interaction provides a repulsive force that drives ions through the skin.

Applied electric current: Electric current alters the molecular arrangement of skin component. This alteration could yield some change in the skin permeability.

'Flipflop' gating: When an electric current is applied across a cellular membrane parallel rearrangement of polypeptides occurs. Pores are thus, opened up as a result of the repulsion between neighboring dipoles and water molecule and ions will flow in the pore channel to neutralize the dipole moments. This phenomenon should lead to an enhancement in skin permeability for peptide and protein molecules and other charged molecules.

Electroosmosis/Convective force: Electroosmosis produces bulk motion of solvent that carries ions or neutral molecules with the solvent stream. The skin is negatively charged at pH values above 4, implying that positively charged ions like Na^+ ions will be more easily penetrated as they attempt to neutralize the charge in the skin to maintain electroneutrality. Thus, the transfer of ions under physiological conditions is from the anode to the cathode. For loss of each cation (sodium ion) from the electrode in this process, a counter ion, i.e., an anion, Cl^- moves in the opposite direction from the cathode to the anode.

Transport number of ion: Which describes the fraction of the total current transmitted by the ion and depends on the physicochemical properties of the respective ions. Na^+ is greater than Cl^- and also the skin facilitates movement of Na^+ more than Cl^-, hence, there is a net increase in the NaCl in the cathodal segment and net decrease in NaCl on the anodal side. Due to this electrochemical gradient, osmotic flow of water is induced from the anode to the cathode. If any neutral drug molecules are present at the anode at this time they can be convicted through the skin along with the water. Such water movement often results in pore shrinkage at the anode and pore swelling at the cathode.

Concentration gradient: Concentration gradient and electrochemical gradient developed across the skin also enhances the drug transport.

Shunt pathway theory: The shunt pathway theory suggests that during iontophoresis, drugs are introduced through the skin by way of glands follicles and/or imperfections in the skin structure.

FACTORS AFFECTING PENETRATION

Charge: Monovalent molecules could be delivered more easily than divalent ones, even if they had similar molecular weight.

Molecular size: As small molecules are more mobile than large molecules hence, they are easily transported.

Solubility: More soluble drugs are easily penetrated.

Ionic strength: If buffer ions are included, they compete with the drug for the delivery, decreasing the quantity of drug delivered.

Viscosity: The migration of drug is inversely related to the viscosity.

Physiological factors: Physiological factors which involves the skin on which the electrode is placed. Factors like its thickness presence or absence of pores, its permeability affects the iontophoretic transport. Sweat glands are most significant route for the conduction of electric charge into the skin.

Amplitude: The rate of penetration is directly proportional to the amplitude of this current. Once it penetrates drug ions will form a reservoir within the avascular epidermal layer just under active electrode. Drug absorption from the reservoir to surrounding tissues occurs by diffusion not the amplitude of the current. If blood vessels under the active electrode are dilated (with higher intensities), drug penetration depth is reduced due to increased clearance.

EFFECTS

Effects can be phoretic, electrolytic, and pharmacological. Phoretic takes place due to the capacity of electrical current to push drug ions through the skin's layer. Electrolysis is the decomposition of a compound by passing direct electrical current through it which leads to electrochemical reactions under electrodes. There will be net accumulation of hydrogen ion under anode and hydroxyl ions under the cathode. This acidic reaction (sclerotic) under anode tends to harden the skin through protein coagulation and alkaline reaction under cathode (sclerolytic) tends to soften the skin through protein liquefaction. This sclerolytic reaction is responsible for erythema of skin and itching and burning sensation under anode. The pharmacological reaction is due to specific effects of a particular drug.

INSTRUMENTATION

Device can be portable, cabinet or a battery embedded wireless device.

Source of current is plain DC.

Electrodes labelling: One larger electrode and other smaller electrode both are separated by 6 inch apart. The ideal distance is the diameter of the largest electrodes. The electrode used for therapeutic effect is called as active electrode or delivery electrode and other electrode is called as dispersive electrode or return electrode.

Types of electrode: The two types are custom made and commercial made (patch type)(Table 41.1).

Custom electrode: It is made up of malleable skin materials with gauze impregnated with therapeutic ionic solution.

Commercial electrode: It is made up of gel matrix or fiber patch impregnated with therapeutic ionic solution.

Table 41.1: Types of electrodes advantages and disadvantages

Electrode	*Advantages*	*Disadvantages*
Custom electrodes	• Low cost • Can be cut into desired shape	• More preparation time • Acidic under anode and alkaline under cathode • Requires straps • Leaking of solution

Contd.

Contd.

Commercial electrodes	• Incorporated with buffering system so no acidic or alkaline changes under electrodes • Predetermined sizes so no preparation time • Cleaner to use, no leakage • Self adhesive	• High cost • Not available in desired shape

PROCEDURE (Described in Chapter 40)

- **Pre-application task**
- **Preparation of apparatus**
- **Prepare the patient psychologically**
- **Prepare the patient physically**
- **Position the patient**
- **Preparation of electrode (described below)**
- **Placement of electrodes (described below)**

Preparation of Electrode

Choose the appropriate electrode custom or commercial. A commercial is preferred over custom as it minimises skin irritation and burn. Apply no weight over electrodes as it increases tissue pressure which increases the chemical burn. Assure a polarity match between drug ion and the electrode polarity. If ion is positively charged keep under anode and if ion is negatively charged keep under cathode

Electrode placement: The active electrode is always placed immediately over the treated area and return electrode is placed far from active electrode. Assure even contact between electrodes and skin to ensure optimal ion delivery into treated area.

End of Treatment

Carefully remove the electrodes and immediately inspect the exposed skin areas for adverse reactions. Apply soothing skin lotion after treatment as it can reduce skin irritation post therapy

DOSIMETRY

Dosimetry depends on following parameters:

Drug selection: See Table 41.2 to different drugs used in iontophoresis its effects and indications. Selection is based on specific therapeutic effect.

Drug ion polarity: Negatively charged ions placed under cathode and positively charged ions placed under anode.

Drug concentration: Drug concentration used for iontophoresis usually range within 2–5% aqueous solution or ointment.

Table 41.2: Commonly used ions in the iontophoresis technique

Sl. No.	*Name of ions*	*Compound*	*Charge*	*Effect*	*Use*	*Solution*
1	Iodine ion	Potassium iodide	Negative	Irritating effect on superficial sensory nerve ending, Increase vasodilatation sclerolytic agent	Chronic inflammatory lesion, softening of superficial scar adhesive capsulitis trigger finger	4.7% Iodex ointment Or 1–10%
2	Chloride ion	Sodium chloride	Negative	Irritating effect on superficial sensory nerve ending, Increase vasodilatation, Sclerolytic agent	Chronic inflammatory lesion, softening of superficial scar Keloid and burns	2% aqueous solution
3	Salicylate ion	Sodium salicylate, Methyl salicylate (iodex ointment), Trolamine salicylate (myoflex ointment)	Negative	Reduce inflammation and pain inhibiting the synthesis of prostaglandin	Rheumatoid arthritis, Rheumatic osteoarthritis Frozen shoulder, Scar tissue Warts	2% aqueous sodium salicylate 4.7% Iodex 10% Trolamine sulphate
4	Albuci ion	Sodium sulphacetamide	Negative	Destroy certain bacteria	Treatment of infection of the eyes	1-5%
5	Acetate ion	Acetic acid	Negative	Remove Ca deposits by sclerolytic action	In case of calcified tendinitis, Myositis ossificans	2% acetic acid
6	Dexamethasone Or Prednisolone Or Triamcinolone	Dexamethasone phosphate (decadron) Methyl prednisolone Triamcinolone diacetate	Negative	Reduces inflammation, Inhibits biosynthesis of prostaglandins	All kinds of Arthritis	0.4%
7	Citrate	Potassium citrate	Negative	Analgesic	Rheumatoid arthritis	2%
8	Diclofenac	Diclofenac sodium	Negative	Reduces inflammation, Inhibits biosynthesis of prostaglandins	Anti-inflammatory Pain relief	0.5–1%
9	Ketoprofen	Ketoprofen sodium	Negative	Reduces inflammation, Inhibits biosynthesis of prostaglandins	Anti-inflammatory Pain relief	10–30%
10	Zinc ion	Zinc sulphate or Zinc chloride or Zinc oxide	Positive	The ion react with the tissue protein to form zinc albucinate which forms a filling over the surface and adhere to underlying tissue, bactericidal effect prevent entry of bacteria	Infected superficial wound, sinus, mucus membrane, for destroying granulation of wound, infection of ear	20% zinc oxide
11	Copper ion	Copper sulphate	Positive	Reduces sensitivity of nasal mucus membrane, Bluish green Copper albucinate is formed	Used in allergic rhinitis or hay fever, fungal infection, sinusitis, dermatophytosis or athletes foot treatment of wound	2% copper sulphate
12	Histamine	Histamine dihydrochloride	Positive	Triple response, Dilation of capillaries by direct effect of histamine, Dilation of arteioles by axonal reflex, Exudation of fluid	Raynaud's disease, Rheumatic condition, Rheumatoid and osteoarthritis, post traumatic fibrositis, Tennis elbow, softening the scar	1% solution

Contd.

Contd.

13	Hyaluronidase	Wydase crystals	Positive	Same effects, but less general effect (effect confined to area of application) increases permeability in connective tissue hydrolysation of hyaluronic acid	For swelling in case of OA and RA lymphedema	Delivered after reconstitution with 0.9% sodium chloride (normasol) to give 150 micro-gram/mL
14	Lidocaine	Lidocaine with epinephrine ion (fraction of 1: 50%)	Positive	Local anesthesia reduces pain by blocking pain transmission	In case of pain and periarthritis bursitis, tendinitis tic doloreux TMJ pain	5% xylocaine ointment Or 2–5%
15	Magnesium	Epsom salt (Magnesium sulphate)	Positive	Muscle relaxation and vasodilation	Wound, spasm, Raynaud's disease	2% aqueous
16	Calcium	Calcium chloride	Positive	Stabilize excitable membranes Decreases excitability threshold in peripheral nerves and skeletal muscle	Muscle spasm Hypersensitive peripheral nerve	2–5% aqueous
17	Hydrocortisone	Hydrocortisone	Positive	Inhibit the biosynthesis of prostaglandin	Used in RA and OA	0.5% ointment
18	Lithium	Lithium chloride Lithium carbonate	Positive	Exchange ion	Gouty typhi and hyperuricemia	2% aqueous solution
19	Priscoline	Benzoline hydrochloride	Positive	Accelerate healing	Indolent ulcers	2% aqueous
20	Tolazoline	Tolazoline hydrochloride	Positive	α-adrenergic receptor antagonist Vasodilator stimulates tissue healing via inhibiting smooth muscle contraction	Ulcers (open wounds)	2% aqueous
21	Glycopyrronium	Glycopyrronium Bromide	Positive	Anticholinergic (reduce sweating)	Hyperhydrosis	0.05%
22	Poldine	Poldine methosulfate	Positive	Anticholinergic (reduce sweating)	Hyperhydrosis	
23	Mecholyl	Derivative of acetylcholine	Positive	Powerful vasodilator, good muscle relaxant and analgesic	Used with discogenic low back radiculopathies and sympathetic reflex dystrophy	0.25% ointment
24	Baclofen	Baclofen solutiom	Positive	Relaxes muscle spasm	Muscle spasm	0.5–2%
25	Water	Tap water	Positive/ Negative	Antisudation/Antisweating by inducing the formation of keratin plugs in the lumen of sweat glands	Hyperhydrosis	100% Use 2X hand baths Reverse polarity halfway through treatment (15+15 minutes)
26	Ringer's solution	Sodium chloride, potassium chloride, calcium chloride and sodium bicarbonate	Positive/ Negative	Cumulative effects of sodium potassium calcium and chloride ions	Open decubitus solution	100%

Dose: The dose is proportional to the current magnitude used and the total application duration.

Recommended current density: *For cathode:* 0.5 mA/cm^2, *For anode:* Not more than 1 mA/cm^2.

Amplitude: Not more than 40 mA/min current density.

Treatment Time

If intensity of 4 mA not more than 10 minutes.

If intensity of 2 mA not more than 20 minutes.

If intensity of 1 mA not more than 40 minutes.

ADVANTAGES

- No skin puncture, it can avoid painful needle injection.
- Avoid the risk of infection from non-sterilized technique.
- Avoids the risk and inconveniences of parenteral therapy, Bypasses liver and GI system thereby avoiding systemic side effects.
- Delivery of ionized as well as unionized molecules.
- Easy termination of drug delivery in case of toxicity.
- Offering better control over the quantity of drug delivered since the amount of drug delivered depends on applied current, duration of applied current and area of skin exposed to the current.
- Prevent variation in the absorption and metabolism as seen with oral administration.
- Reducing significantly inter and intraindividual variability since the rate of drug delivery is more dependent on applied current than on stratum corneum characteristics.
- Utilization of drug candidate with short biological half life and narrow therapeutic index.
- Decreases the total dose and dosing frequency.
- Restoration of the skin barrier property without producing severe skin irritation.
- Facilitate continuous or pulsatile delivery of drug (depending on the current applied).
- Enhancing the delivery of polar molecules as well as high molecular weight compounds.
- Simple non-invasive administration and improved bioavailability.
- Enhanced safety, efficacy, reliability and acceptability.

DISADVANTAGES

- Cannot deliver drug by iontophoresis if drug causes irritation.
- The exact dose may not reach the target.
- There is a limit to the amount of medication that can be delivered usually 5 to 10 mg/hr (time consuming).
- Some drugs cause long lasting pigmentation or erythema formation after iontophoretic application.
- During iontophoretic transport across the skin, the drug encounters potential of hydrogen (pH) differences between 4 and 7.3, leading to the possibility of the drug molecule becoming uncharged and losing the major effect of electric field.

- Formation of Galvanic rash.
- Increasing the current strength or applications for longer periods can lead to pain, burning sensation, blister formation and skin necrosis.
- Iontophoresis is not suggested for under arm or facial/head hyperhydrosis.
- Iontophoresis cannot achieve high drug level in blood.
- Diseased skin as well as extent of disease can affect penetration.
- The metabolic enzyme in the skin can increase the problem.
- Iontophoresis is restricted to drugs that can be formulated in ionized form.
- DC current can cause mast cell to synthesize histamine which cause increase dots all over the skin.

INDICATIONS

- **Hyperhydrosis**
- **Tendinitis:** Supraspinatus tendinitis, Bicipital tendinitis, Achilis tendon, Epicondylytis–Tennis elbow patellar tendinitis, Golfer's elbow, Peyronie's disease.
- **Arthritis:** Osteoarthritis, Rheumatoid arthritis, Gouty arthritis, TM joint arthritis, Post-surgical hip pain, Chronic inflammatory lesions.
- **Scar:** To soften the superficial scar, Infected superficial wound or ulcer, Infections of ear and eyes.
- **Vascular disorders:** Raynaud's disease.
- **Dermatological:** Fungal infection and different skin conditions, plantar warts.
- **Other musculoskeletal:** Plantar fasciitis, Edema, Myofascial syndrome, Myositis ossificans, Myopathy, Post-herpetic neuralgia, Sub-deltoid bursitis, Spasm, RSD.

Contraindications, precaution and danger are same as that of DC detailed in Chapter 37.

42

Sinusoidal Current

DEFINITION

It is an evenly alternating low frequency current with less voltage.

PULSE CHARACTERISTICS

- Sine wave 100 pulses
- 50 Hz; each phase duration is 10 ms, 50 pulse in one direction and 50 pulse in other direction Figure 42.1.
- Voltage 60–80 volt.

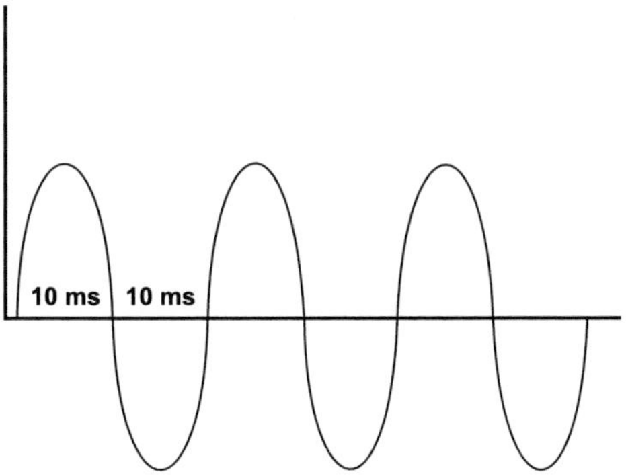

Fig. 42.1: Waveform of sinusoidal current

PRODUCTION

Sinusoidal current can be obtained by reducing the voltage with a step down transformer. As current is bidirectional no rectifier is used. The parts are mentioned below:

Parts

- Step down transformer
- Potential divider
- Surge with a help of valve circuit
- Switch
- Ammeter
- Output electrode
- Two control knobs
  - To increase intensity
  - For changing surge and unsurge
  - No knob to change frequency.

TYPES OF SINUSOIDAL CURRENT

- Surged: Surging is done at the rate of 6–30 surges.
- Unsurged.

Hot Spot

Physiological and therapeutic effects of sinusoidal and faradic currents are same.

PHYSIOLOGICAL EFFECT

1. *Effect on sensory nerve:*
   (a) It irritates sensory nerve; pin prickling sensation and not comfortable for patient.
   (b) Erythema due to vasodilatation.
2. *Effect on motor nerve:* Tetanic contraction.
3. *Effect on denervated muscle:* Not tolerated by the patient.
4. *Effect on muscle tissue:* Rhythmic muscle contraction and relaxation which assist in lymphatic return and venous return.
5. *Chemical effect:* It doesn't have chemical effect since it is a biphasic current.
6. *Effects on tissues of the body:*

   If there is any swelling inflammatory exudate, unsurged sinusoidal current will help the absorption of exudates by channelling the excess fluid to lymphatic and venous tissue. The probable mechanism is because of the alteration in semi-permeability of cell membrane allowing the ions to pass through.
7. *Relief on pain:* Due to the different pain gate theory mechanism and reduction in conduction velocity.

THERAPEUTICS EFFECT

- Pain relief
- Reduction of swelling
- Facilitation of muscle contraction
- Re-education of muscle contraction
- Training a new muscle action
- Neuropraxia
- Severed motor nerve
- Improved venous and lymphatic drainage
- Prevention and loosening of adhesion
- Counter irritation.

INDICATIONS

- **Causalgia (pain along the nerve) due to partial nerve lesion post-herpetic syndrome.**
- **Lymphedema.**
- **And other indications mentioned for faradic currents.**

Contraindications, precautions and dangers are mentioned in Chapter 37.

Burn can occur only with over dose or electrode touching the metal implant.

43

Diadynamic Current

HISTORY

Pierre Bernard. Used in Europe and Australia.

Definition

Diadynamic currents are monophasic sinusoidal current being rectified from main type current.

INSTRUMENTATION AND ELECTRODES

Cabinet type therapeutic stimulator and Surface electrodes with conductive gel as coupling media.

PARAMETERS

Cycle duration and intercycle duration are fixed.

Sine wave frequency in India is 50 Hz, Each phase 10 ms.

PRODUCTION

Electronic modulation of a symmetrical biphasic sinusoidal current.

Frequency is derived from the stimulators own main line power supply of either 50 Hz or 60 Hz.

TYPES

1. **MF: Monophase fixed**

   Half waved rectified sinusoidal current

   Series of 10 ms half sine wave shaped pulse with 10 ms pulse width (Fig. 43.1).

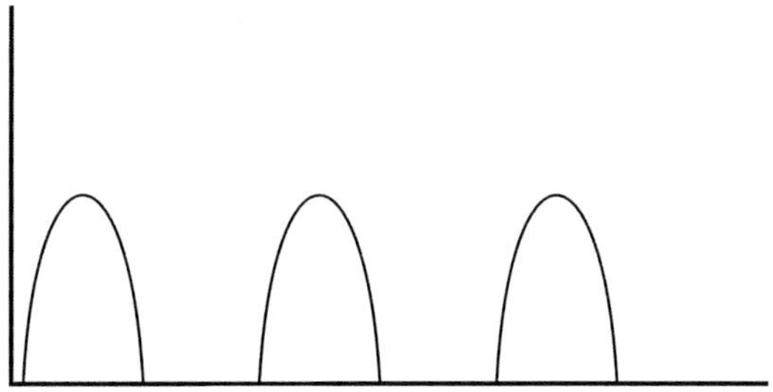

Fig. 43.1: Monophase fixed

2. **DF: Diphase fixed**

   Full wave rectified sinusoidal current.

   Each pulse last for 10 msec and there is no pulse interval (Fig. 43.2).

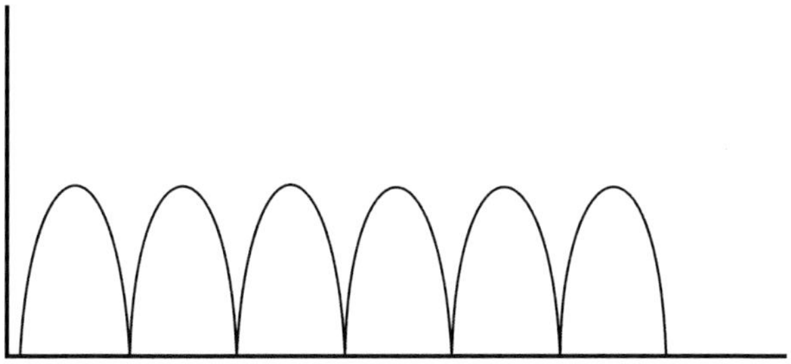

Fig. 43.2: Diphase fixed

3. **CP module : Module en courtes**

   If MF and DF are applied alternately for 1 sec the resulting current is CP module (Fig. 43.3).

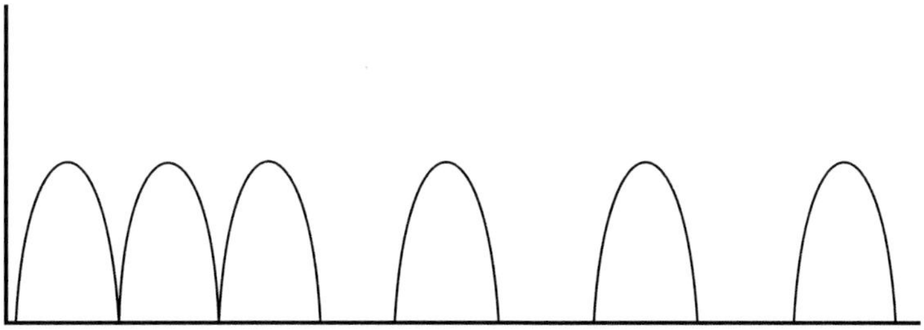

Fig. 43.3: CP module

4. **LP module: Module en longues**

   If 2 MF currents are applied so that one series of pulses occupies the pulse interval of the other, one is of the constant intensity and while other is a surge. Length of each surge is 6 sec (Fig. 43.4).

5. **SRE module: Syncope Rhythm**

Syncope rhythm is one sec of MF followed by 1 sec Rest phase.

Before any of these five applications a low amplitude DC current should be given. This decreases the transmembrane nerve potential, thus minimizing the current amplitude levels associated with the subsequent delivery of any of the modes.

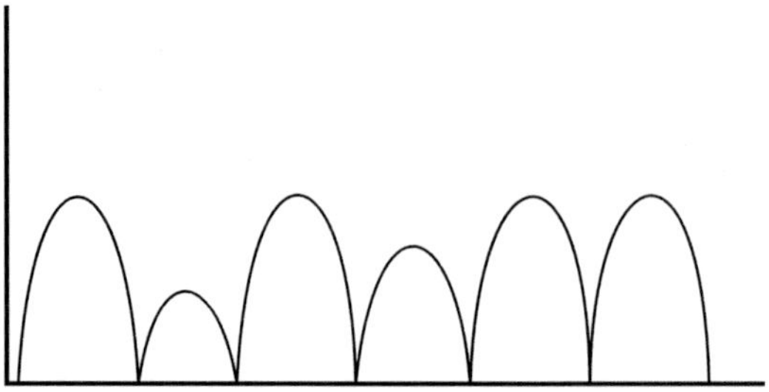

Fig. 43.4

PHYSIOLOGICAL EFFECTS

1. *On Sensory nerve*
   - Pin prickling sensation
   - Erythema
2. *On Motor nerve*

   Tetanic contraction
3. *Edema*

   It alters the autonomic activity by reducing the sympathetic tone
4. *Chemical effect*

   More compared to sinusoidal current
5. *Masking (Fig. 43.5) Or Physiological blocking*

Stimulation

↓

Threshold of nerve is raised

↓

So, sensory nerve doesn't excite

Fig. 43.5: Masking

THERAPEUTIC EFFECTS

1. Relief of pain is obtained through following mechanism:
   - Masking
   - Vasodilatation

- Pain gate theories
- Muscle stimulation which increases blood flow to the muscle

2. Decreased inflammation and swelling due to changes the cell permeability.
3. Muscle re-education and strengthening.
4. Facilitation of tissue healing due to circulatory changes and increased cell activity.

INDICATIONS

1. Any condition with edema.
2. Soft tissue injuries like epicondylitis, contusion.
3. Joint disorders like post-immobilization.
4. Circulatory disorders like Raynaud's disease and migraine.
5. Patellofemoral pain.
6. Peripheral nerve disorders like neuralgia, neuritis, herpes zoster infection, Radiculopathy.
7. Postoperative illeus.

DOSIMETRY

Prior to application of diadynamic current (DC) should be given for three minutes, then an episode of diaphase fixed (DF) followed by a combination of MF, CP, LP, RS.

The purpose of giving DC is to reduce sensitivity which further reduces transmembrane potential of the membrane.

For example, Begin with DC three minutes, then DF two minutes, then MF three minutes, then CP one minute.

Amplitude is set between threshold of perception and threshold of pain.

METHOD OF APPLICATION OF DIADYNAMIC CURRENT

1. *Pain spot application:*
   (a) Anode over the pain spot, cathode adjacent to it; OR
   (b) Cathode proximal in the lymph or over the nerve root supplying the peripheral area and anode over pain spot.
2. *Nerve trunk application:*
   (a) Where the nerve is superficial the electrodes are applied.
3. *Para-vertebral application:*
   (a) Both electrodes to the side of the spine at the level of nerve root supplying the painful area.
4. *Vasotrophic application:*
   (a) Used in case of vascular disorders.
5. *Electrodes are placed along the affected regions:*
   - Myoenergetic application
     (i) One at each end of the muscle belly
     (ii) One on the motor point and other on the proximal point.
   - Trans regional application.

   To treat a joint, electrodes are positioned on the opposite side of the joint.

DOSAGES

1. *Intensity*

   Patient should feel a mild vibration or pricking sensation.

   Treatment time; 10–12 minutes.

2. *Type of Diadynamic current used*

   MF

   Treatment of pain without spasm.

   The patient will feel vibratory sensation.

   Muscle contraction at lower intensity.

   DF

   Used for circulatory condition, acute condition.

   Muscle contraction occurs with higher intensity.

   Point feels prickling sensation.

   CP-Module

   Used for treatment of post-traumatic patient.

   Patient should feel fine tremor and vibration.

   LP-Module

   Used for long-lasting analgesic effect in case of myalgia, neuralgia.

   SR-Module

   Used in conditions where faradic currents are used.

44

High Voltage Pulsed Galvanic Stimulation (HVPGS)

HISTORY

Haslip, developed in 1940 and used in US.

DEFINITION

Twin peak current with high peak intensity but lower average current and very short pulse duration developed from interrupted direct current.

INSTRUMENTATION

Cabinet or portable.

PULSE CHARACTERISTICS

- Developed from interrupted DC.
- High voltage 150–500 volts.
- Pulse duration: 5–200 microseconds.
- Frequency is 2–100 Hz, 30–50 Hz is used for muscle contraction.
- Peak intensity: 2–2.5 Ampere, Average: 1.2–1.5 mA.
- Shape and duration of pulse is fixed. Two types of shape are commonly used (Figs. 44.1A and B).
- Waveform characteristics are detailed in Figure 44.2.

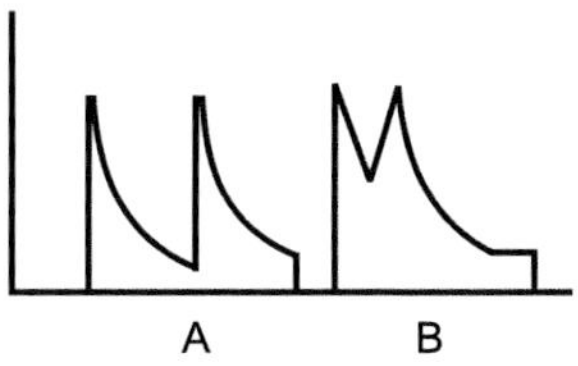

Fig. 44.1: Types of HVPGS pulse (twin peak pulse)

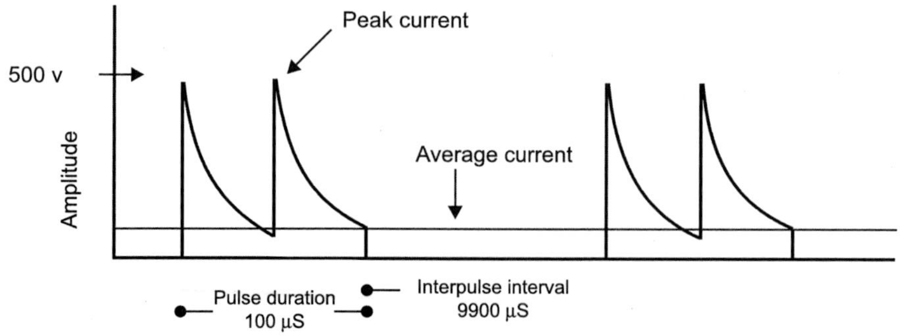

Fig. 44.2: Waveform characteristics of HVPGS

ADVANTAGE

- Since the current is brief in duration, it is easily passed through skin and penetration is deep.
- Because of the discrimination between sensory, motor and pain fibers, the currents are relatively comfortable.
- Less chemical effects compared to faradic currents can apply up to 60 minutes, safe and comfortable up to faradic currents.

DISADVANTAGE

HVPGS cannot stimulate denervated muscles as it cannot depolarize muscle membrane.

TECHNIQUE

- There is no control knob for shape of pulse/duration of pulse.
- Knobs available are – one for intensity, one for frequency, one for intra pulse interval, last one to change the type of HVPGS.

TYPES

- **Continuous mode:** A series of twin pulses delivered continuously.
- **Reciprocal mode:** It refers to alternate application of series of pulse to one or other of the two electrode. It doesn't mean that current direction is reversed.
- **Surged mode:** Intensity is gradually increased.

PHYSIOLOGICAL AND THERAPEUTIC EFFECT

- **Relief of pain:**
  - Due to pain gate theories

  - Stimulating A δ, block C: Low frequency is set, high intensity is given with a small electrode.
  - Stimulating A β blocks A δ: High frequency is set, intensity is less with a big electrode to produce sensory stimulation.
- o Increase blood flow: Removes waste products and debris.

- **Increase joint mobility due to following mechanism:**
  1. Reduction of pain.
  2. Direct effect on blood vessel (Vasodilatation).
  3. Sympathetic stimulation causes vasodilatation. Vasodilatation removes waste products, debris and vasoactive agents.
  4. Reduction of post-traumatic edema (explained in relief of edema).
- **Muscle contraction:**
  - o Increases the movement thereby increases circulation.
- **Relief of oedema due to following mechanisms:**
  - o Muscle pumping effect assisting venous circulation.
  - o **Fluid repulsion theory:** This effect is caused by repulsion under the cathode of negatively charged albumin proteins found in the blood causing a fluid shift and thus, reducing edema at electrode site which is called as fluid repulsion theory.
- **Antispasmodic effect:**

  This is caused inducing muscle fatigue due to prolonged motor unit recruitment leading to muscle exhaustion. Thus, breaks muscle spasm pain cycle. This physiological effect is used in Levator ani syndrome (chronic anal spasm).
- **Wound healing:**

  It accelerates different phases of wound healing through different mechanism explained under Chapter 32 acceleration of wound healing.
- **Electrochemical changes:**

  With HVPGS, since it is a ultrashort pulse duration it does not produce unwanted side effect under electrodes. However, when applied continuously over a long period of time, it can induce skin irritation and burns can occur under the electrodes.

DOSIMETRY

Pulse characteristics as already described. Treatment is given for 30 to 90 minutes, daily 5–7 times a week.

ELECTRODE TYPES

Commercial reusable electrodes are used:

- For dermal wounds: Carbon rubber electrode, Home made aluminium foil.
- For pelvic floor muscle spasm: Intravaginal, intrarectal.

ELECTRODE POLARITY

Since the phases of wound healing overlaps each other periodic reversal of current polarity is required. The automatic current polarity reversal leads to equal periods of cathodal and anodal stimulation of wound site per treatment session. Another way is to alternate between cathode and anode at wound site every three days for entire treatment.

INDICATIONS

- Wound healing
  - Dermal wounds
  - Pressure ulcer
  - Diabetic ulcer
  - Burn wound.
- Post traumatic
  - Edema due to fracture
  - Sprain
  - Strain.
- Musculoskeletal
  - Chronic low back pain
  - Neck pain
  - Delayed onset muscle soreness
  - Wrist pain.
- Levator ani syndrome
- Bell's palsy.

Contraindications, dangers and precautions are mentioned in Chapter 37.

SPECIAL PRECAUTIONS

- Risk of cross contamination in case of wounds and pelvic floor muscle spasm management. In order to prevent cross contamination; (1) wear protective gowns, gloves and mask, (2) discard waste, such as used coupling media, gauze, disposable electrodes in bio-waste bucket.
- Coupling media should be warmer than the wound surface otherwise slows down the mitotic activity which in turns delays wound healing.

Hot Spot

Q. Why HVPC is more effective in edema management compared to other currents?

Ans: It relieves edema due to four mechanisms:

1. Muscle contractions which has a pumping effect which increases venous and lymphatic return.
2. Fluid repulsion theory: as explained before.
3. Removal of vasoactive agents, debris and waste products from the injured area.
4. Increase in cell membrane permeability allowing more extracellular fluid to be reabsorbed.

45

Russian Currents

HISTORY

Russian Physiologist Yakov Kots.

DEFINITION

Time modulated in the form of bursts of electrical cycles of a continuous alternating sine wave current with a carrier frequency of 2500 Hz.

INSTRUMENTATION

Portable or cabinet line powered.

Electrodes: Carbon rubber electrode or pliable stainless steel Knit Fabrics.

Coupling media: Electrode gel.

PULSE CHARACTERISTICS (Fig. 45.1)

Each burst is 10 milli seconds

Interburst = 10 milli seconds

50 burst per seconds

Each burst 25 biphasic symmetrical sinusoidal cycles

Duration of each sine wave in a burst is 400 microsec

Half sine wave is 200 micro sec

A 10 milli seconds burst = 25 cycles.

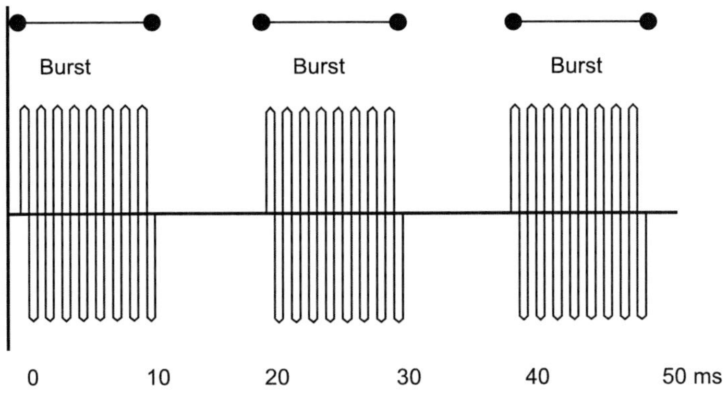

Fig. 45.1: Pulse characteristics of Russian currents

RATIONALE

Compare to other NMES, Russian currents are painless current. Since it is a medium frequency current, it produces no sensory discomfort during maximal evoked muscle tetanic contraction. Since it is painless, higher current amplitude can be delivered to the soft tissues so that deeper motor nerve fibers can be activated. This results in depolarization of Type IIa and IIb muscle fibers thereby increasing the magnitude of electrically evoked tetanic contraction. Overall, it helps in increasing the muscle strength in healthy people.

PHYSIOLOGICAL AND THERAPEUTIC EFFECTS

By the application of Russian currents, there will be depolarization of the nerves which results in motor unit activation. This depolarization depends on burst frequency not the total number of pulses within each burst. The current amplitude determines the force of contraction. The motor unit activation depends on spatial and temporal recruitment. Spatial MU recruitment depends on number and type of fibre activated. The number refers to amount or percentage and order refers to sequence of activation based on size of each MU, i.e., from slow twitch to fast twitch fibers. This is known as Henneman size principle of MU activation. With the stimulation the order is reversed, i.e., from larger (fast twitch) to smaller (slow twitch). Temporal MU recruitment refers to rate of discharge or frequency with which motor units are recruited. It is also called as rate coding. For example, a given MU may be activated several times per second while another MU may be activated a few times per second. With electrical stimulation MU are activated synchronously. The activation of motor units results in tetanic contraction which results in muscle fiber hypertrophy (trophic mechanism) and muscle strengthening.

PARAMETERS AND DOSIMETRY

Current amplitude: Adjust the level to 40–60% MVC.

Burst frequency: 50 Burst per sec.

ON:OFF time ratio: This ratio is defined as the time during which the muscle is activated to the time muscle is not activated, normally set as 10s:50s.

Duty cycle: Once the ON:OFF time ratio is set then duty cycle is automatically set. For the above, e.g., 10s:50s, duty cycle is (10/10 + 50) * 100 = 16.7%.

Ramp up and ramp down: This setting makes electrically induced muscle contraction to mimic voluntary contraction. It is set for 1–2 seconds.

Electrode placement: Monopolar, bipolar, quadripolar or multipolar.

Electrode orientation: Each pair is arranged parallel not perpendicular to the direction of muscle fibers so that it is at the estimated line of pull of the muscle.

Time delay switch: With this stimulation mode, it can be synchronous, reciprocal or overlap mode. *In synchronous mode,* both channels are triggered simultaneously. This is achieved by not setting the time delay. *In reciprocal mode,* when channel one is on, channel two is off and vice versa. This can be achieved by setting time delay equal to on time of channel one. *In overlapping mode,* when channel two overlaps with on time and off time of channel one. This can be achieved by setting time delay more than one second but less than the on time of channel one.

PROCEDURE

Training method can be stimulation alone or in combination with voluntary contraction. In combination method electrical stimulation is superimposed on a given level of voluntary muscle contraction. Maximum 10 contractions are given in each bout. Each bout is separated by 5 minutes rest period. 3–5 bouts can be given at a time.

INDICATIONS

Muscle weakness due to:

- Posterior or anterior ACL reconstruction.
- Total knee replacement.
- Bell's palsy.
- Knee osteoarthritis.
- Patellofemoral syndrome.
- Post-knee sprain muscle atrophy.

Contraindications, dangers and precautions are given in Chapter 37.

46

Rebox Current

HISTORY

Petr Slovak, 1970 Czechoslovakia.

The name Rebox is derived from the 'Rehabilitation Box'.

DEFINITION

Rebox electrotherapeutic method is based on non-invasive transcutaneous application of medium frequency electric currents to a living tissue. Main indications for using the Rebox include treatment of acute and chronic pain, immobility, musculoskeletal and neurological disorders and edema. The currents are introduced transcutaneously to the affected region with a touch of a small non-invasive treatment electrode (cathode) while the patient holds a second reference electrode (anode) in a hand to complete electric circuit.

PULSE CHARACTERISTICS

Battery powered.

Shape of the pulse: Rectangular

Frequency: 2–4 KHz

Pulse width: 100–300 μS

Amplitude: 100–200 μA

Dosage

The treatment electrode (active surface 1.5 mm^2) is applied for 2–3 seconds in one spot, then proceeding approx. 1.5 cm to another point. About 20 points are treated per one session. Frequency of treatment sessions is individual for each patient.

DEVICE DESCRIPTION

Amplitude button: To increase amplitude.

Meter: Average current flowing to the tissue.

Audio output: The intensity of sound output is proportional to the average value of the treatment current. Volume can be controlled by sound button.

Treatment Mode

Gentle mode: Recommended for treating a new patient.

Standard mode: Most frequent mode.

Analgetic mode: To reduce localized hypersensitivity. It is used when a mere touch of probe electrode causes pain.

Electrode Used is Probe Electrode

Cathode: Classic hard tip or Golden flexi tip.

Anode: Cylindrical.

PHYSIOLOGICAL EFFECTS

- Transcutaneous correction of local acidosis (TCLA) described in Table 46.1.
- Local changes in Calcium ions which causes myorelaxation.
- Increased blood circulation and lymphatic circulation.

THERAPEUTIC EFFECTS

1. **Relief of pain:** The main cause of pain is local acidosis due to inflammation and ischemic processes. The mechanism of immediate pain relief is this correction of local acidosis (TCLA) already described.
2. **Reduction of muscle tone, spasm and increased range of motion:** Local changes in calcium ions (Ca^{2+}) concentrations cause myo-relaxation (decrease of muscular hypertonia and spasm) and significant improvement in range of motion.
3. **Neurological disorders:** Rebox therapy is used in rehabilitation of after-stroke conditions, Multiple Sclerosis, phantom pain, Parkinson disease and other conditions.
4. **Healing processes:** The method facilitates healing processes; this effect is mostly visible in wounds after surgery.
5. **Diagnostic purpose:** Tissue electric micro characteristics can be visualized by the Rebox devices. The physiological curve differs from pathological situations and is specific for variety of disorders. This diagnostic value is helpful for monitoring of effectiveness and progress of treatment.

The Normal Physiologic Curve

After 2–3 seconds of needle probe application balance occurs and the current remains constant as shown in the Figure 46.1.

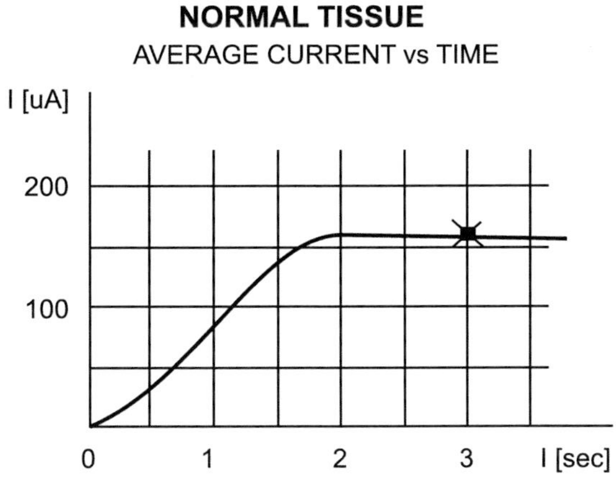

Fig. 46.1: Normal physiologic curve

In Pathological situations, normal shape of the curve changes (Fig. 46.2).

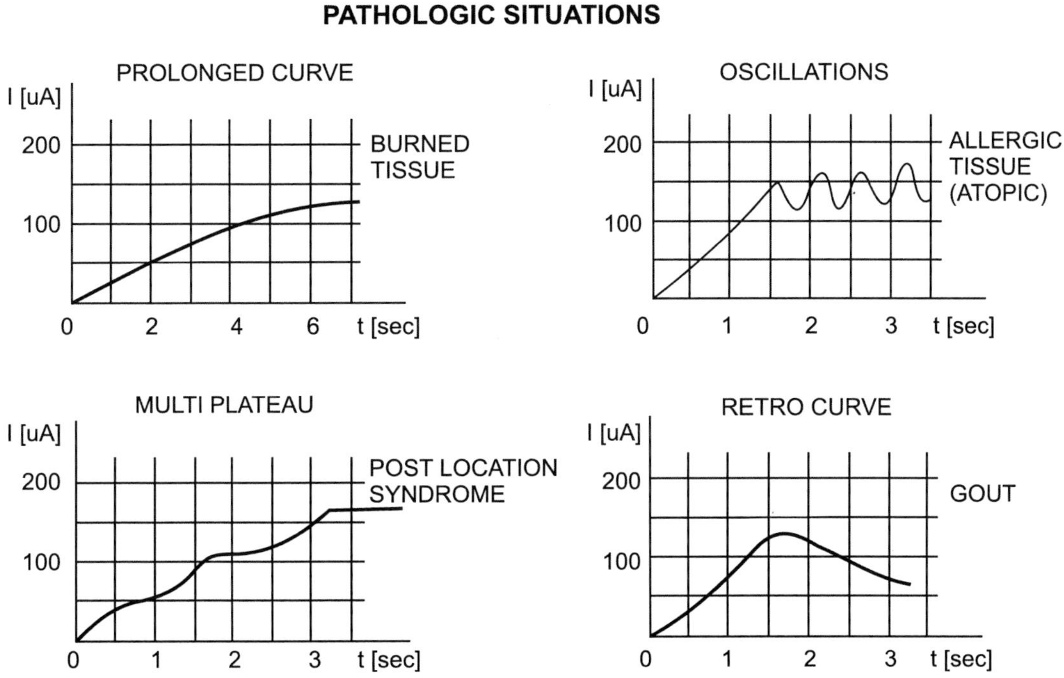

Fig. 46.2: Change of curve in pathologic situations

The therapist receives information from the patient's tissues during treatment, giving him the great advantage of continuous monitoring and control of the dosage applied. Because every type of tissue pathology shows its own specific course of changes in the electric current during treatment, a shape of a displayed curve acts as a diagnostic aid as well as a treatment monitor.

Table 46.1: TCLA

What is Transcutaneous Correction of Local Acidosis – TCLA

The acute injuries and chronic diseases are accompanied by local acidosis due to release of hydrogen ions. This results in pain, myocontraction (spasm) and edema. With Rebox current application, all positive ions (mainly K^+, Ca^{++} and Na^+) are attracted from the extracellular fluid to the cathode. After a short time, myorelaxation in the tissue occurs due to changes in local concentration of calcium ions.

Due to the electrolysis effect, water molecules in extracellular fluid dissociate to hydrogen positive ions and OH hydroxide negative ions according to the chemical equation in the figure. Since hydrogen ions leave the tissue and enter the surrounding air, and hydroxide ions together with K^+ and Na^+ ions create hydroxides NaOH and KOH, local alkalization occurs. This results in dramatic pain decrease. Because the effective radius, which was experimentally found, is about 1.5 cm (approx. 1/2 inch), the treated area for one needle probe application point as a hemisphere with a 1.5 cm radius. There will be improved blood and lymphatic fluid circulation due to increased ion migration (Fig. 46.3).

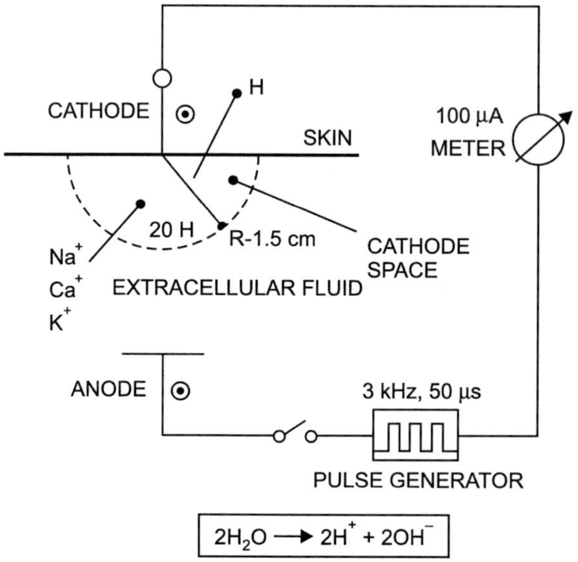

Fig. 46.3: Electrolysis in cathode space

INDICATIONS

1. **Treatment of acute and chronic pain**
   (a) Back pain
   (b) Joint pain
   (c) Pain after injury
   (d) Acute muscle strain
   (e) Osteoarthrosis
   (f) Gouty arthritis

(g) Calcaneal spurs
(h) Post-operative pain

2. **Rehabilitation of Musculoskeletal System**
   (a) Muscle hypertonia and spasms
   (b) Limited joint mobility
   (c) Tendovaginitis
   (d) Bursitis
3. **Antioedematic Effect**
   (a) Swelling treatment
4. **Acceleration of Healing Processes**
   (a) Tendon injury
   (b) Post-operative wounds
5. **Neuro-rehabilitation** (Experimental stage)
   (a) After-Stroke
   (b) Multiple Sclerosis and other conditions.

Contraindications, precautions and dangers are mentioned in Chapter 37. Special care should be taken if the REBOX is used in the neck area of the carotid sinus, to avoid stimulation of the vagus nerve.

47

Micro Currents

SYNONYMS

1. MENS: Micro current Electrical Neuromuscular Stimulator (later the 'N' was removed as the micro amperage current is too weak to stimulate a nerve. Now it is called as 'MES'.
2. Bio stimulation.
3. Micro electrotherapy.

DEFINITION OF MICRO CURRENT

Micro currents can be defined as transcutaneous delivery of continuous and pulsed electrical current wave forms of amplitude with in micro amperage range, i.e., from 1 to 999 μA or less than 1 mA. Micro currents are low voltage current in micro ampere range pulsating between 0.1–680 Hz. The current is too low or weak to produce muscle contraction or to block pain. But its effectiveness is often superior in many application than that of faradic, IFT and TENS. Current is hardly perceptible. It mimics the body own electrical current.

CHARACTERISTICS

Stimulator: Cabinet type in combo mode with other currents and portable type.

Wave form: Constant or pulsed.

Amplitude: Never exceed 1 mA or 1000 μA.

Electrodes: Either carbon impregnated silicon rubber electrodes, fiber electrodes or disposable homemade aluminium foil electrodes.

DIFFERENCE FROM MACRO CURRENTS

The difference is listed in Table 47.1.

Table 47.1: Difference between micro and macro currents

Micro current	Macro current
The current less than range of 300–500 μA	Current greater than 1 mA
Instruments are specialized micro current devices	Instruments are separate for IFT, TENS, Galvanic and faradic
Frequency 0.6–680 Hz	Galvanic → 30 Hz Faradic → 50–100 Hz
Facilitate healing process	Inhibit healing process at higher intensity
Effects takes place at cellular level	Takes place at tissue level

PRINCIPLE OF HEALING BY MICRO CURRENTS

In order to understand the principle of healing, normal concepts should be learned first, i.e., skin battery and current of injury.

Skin battery: Becker hypothesized that a direct current bioelectrical system is present in the human body and that this system is responsible for maintaining tissue health.

Currents of injury: Becker further hypothesized that when the body is injured a disturbance within the body electrical system causes the shift in the current flow at the site of injury, which the author labelled as currents of injury.

Micro current mimics and amplifies those endogenous, weak human skin batteries at the wound site to augment body tissue healing and repair.

Physiology of Injury

- In injured area there is reduction of ATP and causes spasm which leads to reduced oxygen and nutrient to the muscle.
- It also destructs Na^+-K^+ pump.
- Also results in accumulation of metabolic by products.
- All of these events are perceived by point as pain.
- A damage tissue cell produces an electric current through the loss of intracellular ion and destruction of Na^+-K^+ pump mechanism.
- Micro current changes these normal electrical potential neutral so the injured cell attempt to store the normal function to the damaged tissue by normal electrical potential.

PHYSIOLOGICAL EFFECTS

1. Stimulate cellular physiology and growth.
2. Stimulate ATP generation.
3. Re-establishment of Na^+– K^+ pump due to increased mitochondrial function.
4. Increased ability of the cell to synthesize protein.

5. Restoration of polarisation to the tissue.
6. Increased cell permeability.
7. Reduction of inflammatory and exudative process.
8. Acceleration of proliferative and remodelling phases.

THERAPEUTIC EFFECTS

1. Increased rate of collagen function.
2. Accelerate healing of ulcer in the skin.
3. Accelerate wound healing.
4. Accelerate bone fracture healing.
5. Healing of muscle, ligament and tendon injury.
6. Suppression of bacterial growth.
7. Spasmolysis of smooth muscles of circulatory and lymphatic system.
8. Increased tonicity of elastic fiber.
9. Reduction of degeneration process.

Due to above effects the microcurrents overall relieves the pain.

INDICATIONS

Dermal Wounds

Conditions, such as, Epicondylitis, Shoulder Peritendinitis, Trigger points, LBA, TM Joint disorders, Migraine.

DOSIMETRY

Electrode polarity: Anodal stimulation should be used for inflammatory phase and Cathodal stimulation will be used for proliferative and maturative phase. Both can be used for germicidal effect. Since phases of wound healing overlaps it is recommended that polarity should be reversed every three days for the duration of the treatment.

Delivery can be either continuous or pulsed. If it is pulsed, can be applied at 0.1 to 200 pps.

Electrode placement:

For wound: Over the wound or around the wound.

For pain: Over acupuncture point.

For migraine: Through transcranial.

Strength: It depends on the severity of pain and varies from person to person. But not more than 1 mA.

Duration of treatment: 30 to 120 minutes, 1–4 sessions per day, 5–7 days per week.

CONTRAINDICATIONS

1. Epilepsy
2. Pregnant women
3. Cardiac points
4. Points with pacemaker.

ADVANTAGE

1. Non-hazardous
2. Safe for all groups (age)
3. No side effects.

DISADVANTAGE

1. Unpredictable result
2. Time consuming.

48

Pain

DEFINITION

"Pain is defined as unpleasant sensory and emotional experience, i.e., associated with actual or potential tissue damage", according to IASP and Merskey.

CHARACTERISTICS OF PAIN

1. **Threshold and intensity:** If intensity of stimulus is below threshold, pain will not be felt. As intensity increases, more and more pain is felt. According to Webber Fechner's law, $R = \alpha \log S$ where R = Intensity of reaction, S = Intensity of stimulus.
2. **Adaptation:** Pain receptors show no adaptation. Pain continues as long as receptor continues to be stimulated.
3. **Localisation of pain:** Superficial pain is better localized than deep pain.
4. **Emotional:** Pain sensations accompanied by emotions.
5. **Influence of the rate of damage on intensity of pain:** If rate of tissue injury is high, intensity of pain will be high.

REACTIONS OF PAIN

1. **Behavioral:** Expressions, like crying/moaning/frustration/mental/irritation/depression.
2. **Muscular:** Spasm of skeletal muscles in the affected region.
3. **Changes in autonomic nervous system:** Pain is accompanied by signs of sympathetic over activity. For example, rise of BP, tachycardia, pupillary dilation, etc.
4. **Reflex response:** A painful stimulus will be always associated with somatic reflexes. For example, pin prick in the sole of foot leads to withdrawal of foot.

CLINICAL MODELS OF PAIN

1. Acute pain/Chronic pain.
2. Somatogenic pain/Visceral pain.
3. Referred pain/Radiating pain.
4. Psychogenic pain/Neuropathic pain.

   1. **Acute pain:** Acute pain is of recent and sudden onset with demonstrable etiology, and limited course. Function of acute pain is to alert the individual to actual or potential tissue damage so that appropriate measures may be taken, i.e., the withdrawal from the stimulus to prevent further injury (Fig. 48.1).

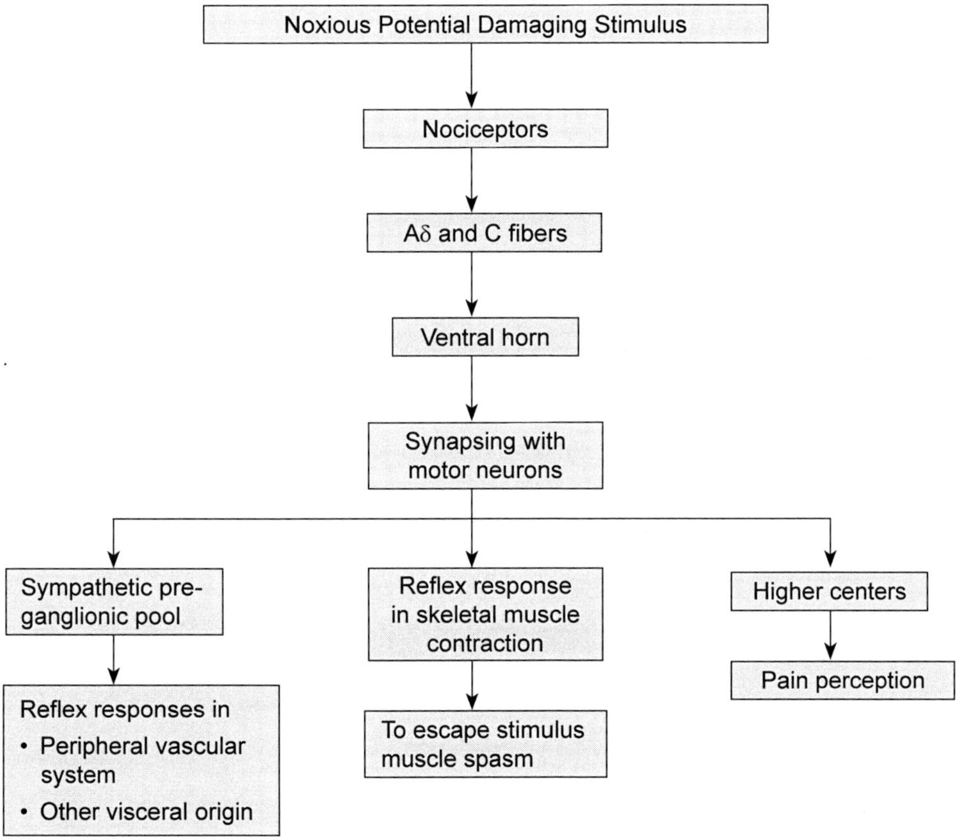

Fig. 48.1 Acute pain

   2. **Chronic pain:** Pain of long duration often associated with anguish, apprehension, depression or hopelessness (Fig. 48.2).

      Causes

      (i) Increase sensitivity of nociceptors.

      (ii) Long lasting peripheral nerve compression.

Compression leads to destruction of large primary afferent neuron as a result, imbalance of large tactile and small (pain) fiber input occurs thereby keeping gate open.

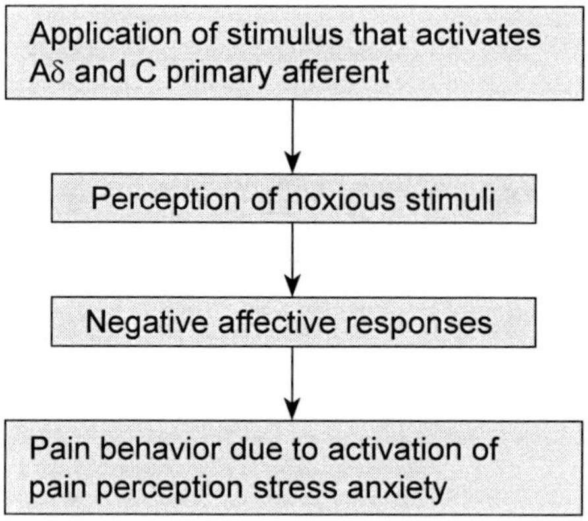

Fig. 48.2: Chronic pain

3. **Somatic and visceral pain:** Somatic pain divides into superficial and deep seated pain

   Visceral pain arises from viscera, it includes:

   (i) Ischemia, e.g., Cardiac pain
   (ii) Obstruction of hollow viscera, e.g., Large intestine
   (iii) Inflammation, e.g., Appendicitis
   (iv) Distension, e.g., Distended bladder
   (v) Severe vasodilation, e.g., Headache.

4. **Referred pain:** Pain felt at the site in the body elsewhere from the source of disease or injury. For example, myocardial infarction, radiating down the left arm.

   Features

   (i) Pain is felt at the dermatome which corresponds to viscerotome of pain producing viscera.
   (ii) Referred pain is felt at an area where the viscera was situated in embryonic life.

Theories of Referred Pain

(i) Convergence theory: Sympathetic afferent fibers carrying same pain sensation emerges from viscera and afferent somatic nerve emerging from the pain receptors of corresponding dermatome of the viscera enters same segment and terminates on the same secondary neurons (Fig. 48.3).

(ii) Subliminal fringe effect: Afferent sympathetic fibers bringing pain sensation from viscera terminates on second order neuron but at the same time also via collateral stimulates another second order neuron. These second order neuron is synapsing with somatic neuron of corresponding dermatome (Fig. 48.4).

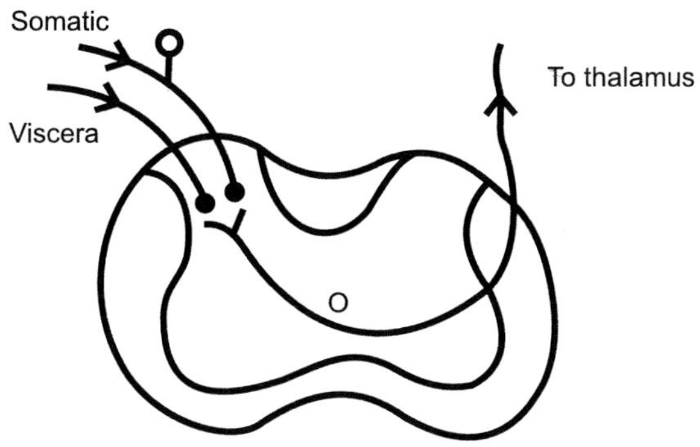

Fig. 48.3. Convergence theory

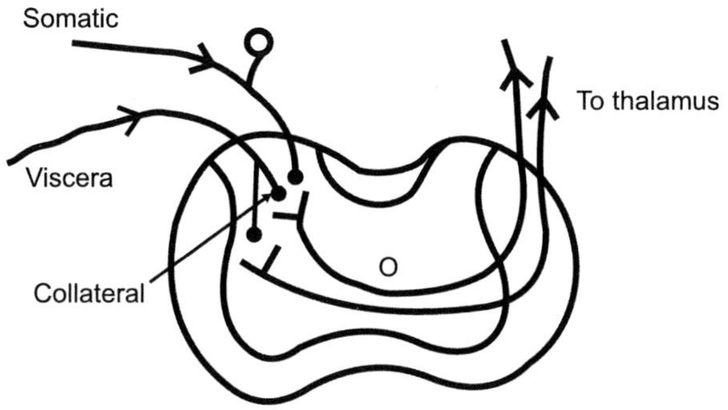

Fig. 48.4: Subliminal fringe effect

NEUROBIOLOGY AND MOLECULAR BIOLOGY OF PAIN

Chemical agents are released as a result of local tissue damage mainly stimulate nociceptors.

1. **Substance that stimulate nociceptors:**
   - (i) Protons (H^+).
   - (ii) Neurotransmitter: 5-hydroxy tryptamine (5 HT or serotonin), Histamine, Acetylcholine.
   - (iii) Polypeptide: Bradykinin, Kallidin.
   - (iv) Prostaglandins.
   - (v) Cellular metabolites: ATP Lactic acid.
   - (vi) Spicy plants: Capaicin (red pepper), Capsicum (black pepper).

   How the substance causes pain?

   - Protons: These are acidic hence, associated with brief depolarization of sensory nerve fibers.
   - 5 HT, ATP and Capaicin: Act directly by opening of ion channels of nociceptive neurons.
   - Bradykinin and Histamine: They act by stimulating a second messenger system.

- Prostaglandins and leucotrines: They act indirectly:
  - Prostaglandins sensitizing the nociceptors to polypeptide bradykinin.
  - Leucotrines act by causing the release of other neuro active agents from polymorphonuclear leucocytes.
- ATP and other metabolites: They release from active cells which stimulate nociceptors directly or indirectly; directly by opening ion channels or indirectly by releasing neuro active agents.
- Red pepper: They activate a specific receptor which depolarises the C fiber to cause brief pain.

2. **Primary afferent neuron:** Substance P: It is the neurotransmitter released at the endings of those primary afferents which originate from somatic structures.

   Vasointestinal peptide: It is released at endings of those primary afferents which originate from visceral structures.

3. **Neurotransmitters in dorsal horn:** At any given synapse more than one transmitter may be involved. Aspartate and Glutamate are excitatory on dorsal horn. Aspartate acts on specific NMDA receptors (N methyl D aspartate) NMDA receptors mediate a phenomenon called wind up in which nociceptive stimulus arriving in the dorsal horn undergo a cumulative increase in the magnitude. This is important mechanism in the explanation of painful areas, i.e., characteristic of clinical chronic pain size. GABA and Glycine are inhibitory neurotransmitters and evidence suggests that GABA is involved in the modulation of nociceptive transmission (Table 48.1).

Table 48.1: Different types of neurotransmitters

Chemical class	*Excitatory*	*Inhibitory*
Amino acid		
Aspartate	+	
Glutamate	+	
GABA		+
GLYCINE		+
Peptides		
Substance P	+	
VIP	+	
Enkaphalin		+
Dynorphin		+

GABA interneuron from the endings of which GABA is released which in turns do presynaptic inhibition. It stops the release of excitatory neuro transmitters from the endings of nociceptive C fibers.

PERIPHERAL AND CENTRAL MECHANISM OF PAIN

1. **Peripheral Mechanism:**

   Receptors: These are free nerve endings, called as nociceptors located in:

   - Cardiac
   - Viscera
   - Skin.

   Stimuli needed are:

   - Intense heat
   - Intense cold
   - Strong mechanical deformation
   - Chemical substances.

   Types

   - **Specific nociceptors:** Those receptors respond to only one noxious stimulus.
   - **Polymodal nociceptors:** Those receptors respond to several noxious stimuli.

   Tissue trauma results in liberation of number of chemical factors from damaged tissue. Chemical factors, such as Substance P-Somatokinin, bradykynin, cholecystokinin, vasoactive peptides, with in primary afferent neurons thought to mediate central pain transmission.

   Primary Afferent Neuron: These are A delta and C fibers. Characteristics are mentioned in the Table 48.2.

Table 48.2: Characteristics of primary afferent neuron

Characteristics	*A delta*	*C fiber*
Type	Group III primary afferent	Group IV afferent
Velocity	Velocity 4–30 m/s	0.5–2 m/s
Type of pain	Sharp and pricking	Burning sensation, more diffusely located
Duration they carry	Short duration	Longer duration
Component	Fast component called as acute pain	Slow component, chronic pain

   Termination in the dorsal horn

   As the primary afferents for pain approach spinal cord they divided into short ascending and descending branches that enter dorsolateral fasciculus, lissauer's tract. A delta (Aδ) and C fibers terminate mainly with in dorsolateral parts of dorsal horn with in lamina I and II. A-delta fibers have also significant input to lamina V of dorsal horn. Nociceptors of skin will terminate in lamina II. Viscera's and muscles will terminate in lamina I and V. Lamina II is largely concerned to localized painful stimuli. Viscera and muscles do not project here may account for diffuse and poorly localized quality of visceral and muscle pain.

2. **Central Mechanisms of Pain:**

   Second Order Neuron

Two major routes by which pain sensations ascend to higher brain centers:

(i) Spinothalamic tract: Pain from Aδ fibers (fast component).

(ii) Spinoreticulothalamic tract – from C fibers (slow component).

Spinothalamic Tract

Axons arising from lamina I and V cross the midline. Run in lateral funiculus as lateral spinothalamic tract conducts through Spinal cord, Medulla, Pons and Midbrain terminate in thalamus.

In thalamus, it terminates as:

(i) Ventral posterolateral nucleus – allows to localize origin of painful stimuli on body surface.

(ii) Posterior complex nuclei – immediate awareness of pain.

(iii) Intra laminar nuclei – emotional and unpleasant aspects of pain.

Spinoreticulothalamic Tract

Neurons give rise to spinoreticulothalamic pathway are located in lamina VII, VIII. These neurons receive their nociceptive input via inter neurons from the areas of grey matter where Aδ and C fibers terminate. Spinoreticulothalamic tract have short axons thus, requiring multiple neurons and synapses and this tract is bilateral. Fibers terminate predominantly in intra laminar nuclei of thalamus.

Pathway for emotional and unpleasant aspects of pain.

Spinothalamic tract cells of dorsal horn can be classified in their response properties into four:

(i) Low threshold units: Responding to light mechanical stimuli, such as light touch.

(ii) Wide dynamic range units: Which evokes pain as well as low intensity stimulation.

(iii) High threshold units: Stimuli that are intense enough to inflict tissue damage and nociceptors.

(iv) Thermo sensitive units: Responding to warming or cooling.

Wide dynamic range cells receive input from multiple sources located in lamina V. These neurons receive large number of afferents, so these second order neurons code action potential. So low frequency of action potential, represent a touch stimulus; higher frequency of action potentials represent a noxious stimuli. These all contribute to localization aspect of pain as well as modality discrimination (Table 48.3).

Table 48.3: Components of pain experience

Aspect	Location
Discrimination	Cortex, Thalamus
Affective	Limbic structures
Autonomic responses	Thalamus, Reticular formation

The third order neuron starts from thalamus and ends in the sensory cortex. A summary of physiology of pain pathway is mentioned in the Figure 48.5.

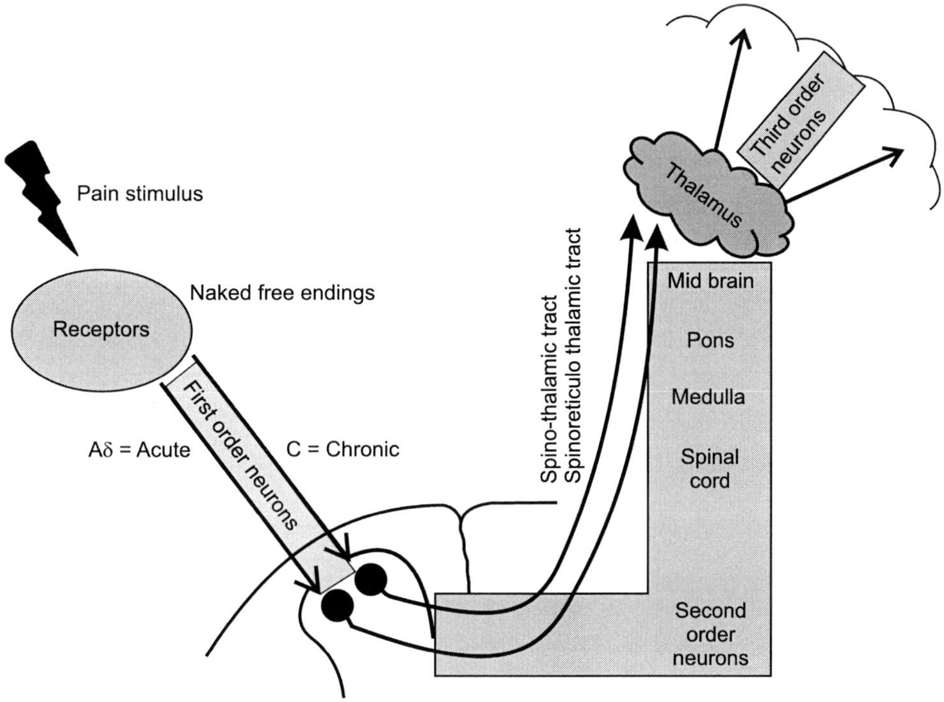

Fig. 48.5: Pain pathway

THEORIES OF PAIN

All the pain theories are described in the Table 48.4. In that pain gate theory will be explained in detail.

Table 48.4: Theories of pain

Sl. No.	*Name of the theory*	*Author/Year*	*Principles*
1.	Intensive summation theory	Erb 1874 Further developed by Goldscheider 1884	Build on Aristotle concept Pain resulted from the excessive stimulation of sense of touch. Describe both stimulus intensity and central summation as clinical determinants of pain.
2.	Strong's theory	Strong 1895	Pain was an experience based on the noxious stimuli and cyclic reactions provoked by the sensations.
3.	Specificity theory	Vonfrey 1895	Receptors will be specific to particular type of sensory experience.
4.	Pattern theory	Nafe 1934	All cutaneous qualities are produced by spatial and temporal patterns of nerve impulses rather than by separate modality specific transmission routes.

Contd.

Contd.

5.	Central summation theory	Livingstone 1943	Intense stimulation resulting from nerve and tissue damage activate fibers that project into Interneuronal pools within the spinal cord.
6.	Fourth theory of pain	Hardly, Wolff, Goodell 1940	The pain was composed of two components: The perception of pain and reaction of it. Reaction was described as complex physio-psychogical process involving cognitive function of individual influence by past experiences, culture and various psychological factors which influence the pain perception.
7.	Sensory interaction theory	Noordenbos 1959	Description of two systems involving transmission of pain and other sensory information, with fast and slow systems. Slow systems (unmyelinated small diameter fibers) were presumed to conduct somatic and visceral afferents. Fast system composed of large fibers were said to inhibit transmission of small fibers.
8.	Gate control theory	Melzack and Wall 1965	Dorsal horn of spinal cord act like a gate that can increase or decrease the flow of nerve impulses, from peripheral fibers to spinal cord cells that project to the brain.

PAIN GATE THEORIES

Pain gate theory was proposed by Melzack and wall. Initially, it consists of three theories. Later Peripheral mechanism was also added to it.

1. Segmental mechanism (Two theories).
2. Extrasegmental mechanism/Descending pain pathway mechanism.
3. Peripheral mechanism.

Segmental Mechanism

1. Stimulation of A-β fibers blocks A-δ fibers at the level of spinal cord. This results in inhibiting acute pain. Thus, acute pain is blocked by stimulation of mechanoreceptors which is carried through A-β fibers. A practical example for this is, if somebody finger gets jammed they immediately blow the air to the hand or they rub the fingers thereby relief was obtained. Here, mechanoreceptors are activated either through vibration or rubbing. As spinal cord allows only one sensation to pass through and mechanoreceptors always bypasses pain sensation, patient obtains the pain relief (Fig. 48.6).
2. Stimulation of A-δ fibers blocks C fibers at the level of spinal cord. This results in inhibiting chronic pain. Thus, chronic pain is blocked by creating acute pain which is carried through A-δ fibers. A practical example for this is, if somebody has long time trapezitis, if someone presses at the same site a immediate relief of trapezitis was obtained. By pressing an acute pain was created which is carried by A-δ fibers. Some of this fibers end in interneurons at dorsal horn in spinal cord

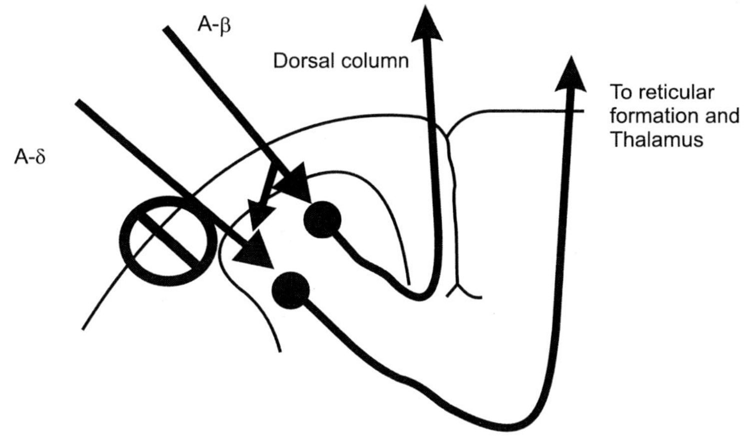

Fig. 48.6: Segmental mechanism theory no. 1

which produces presynaptic inhibition on C fibers. This blocks C fibers and chronic pain relief was obtained (Fig. 48.7).

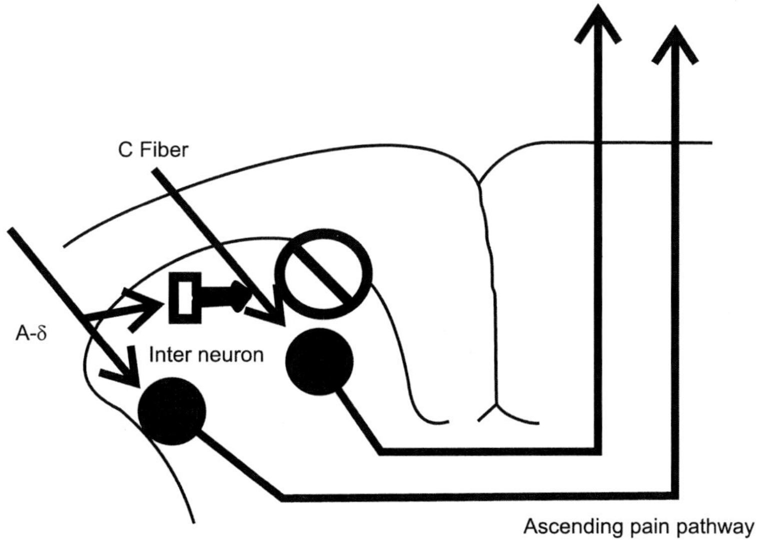

Fig. 48.7: Segmental mechanism theory no. 2

Descending Pain Pathway Mechanism/Extrasegmental Mechanism

By this mechanism C fiber itself block C fiber transmission. Chronic pain is carried by C fibers. The second order neurons travels up to spinal cord which is called as spinoreticulothalamic tract. Some of the collaterals of these tract reaches Peri Aqueduct Grey Matter present in the midbrain and Raphae nucleus in medulla. When collaterals stimulate these areas it activates descending pain pathway which reaches spinal cord. This produces presynaptic inhibition on C fibers. This relieves chronic pain Figure 48.8.

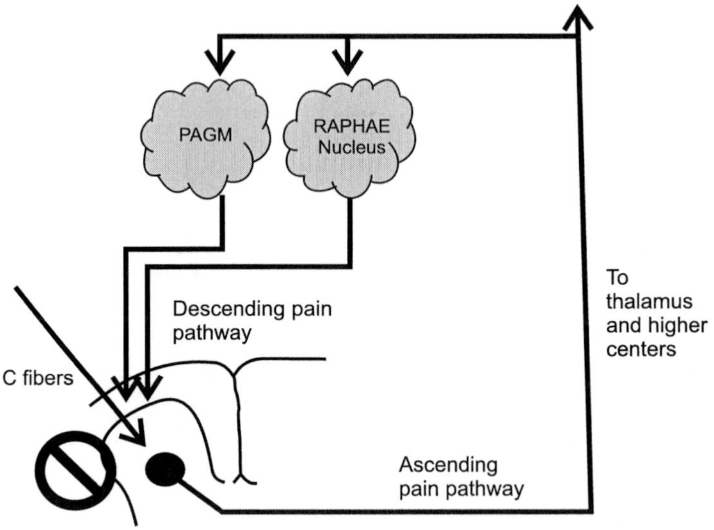

Fig. 48.8: Descending pain pathway

Peripheral Mechanism

The pain impulse travels to spinal cord from a receptor through a sensory nerve. Suppose if TENS electrodes are placed anywhere along the course of the nerve. TENS current produces both orthodromic and antidromic impulses. The antidromic impulses travel towards the receptors stimulated by pain stimulus. They cancel the impulses generated by noxious event.

The orthodromic impulses travel towards brain through spinal cord and thalamus. The patient will feel pain due to the application of TENS stimulus not pain sensation aroused from the pain stimulus site. Thus, it is blocked (Fig. 48.9).

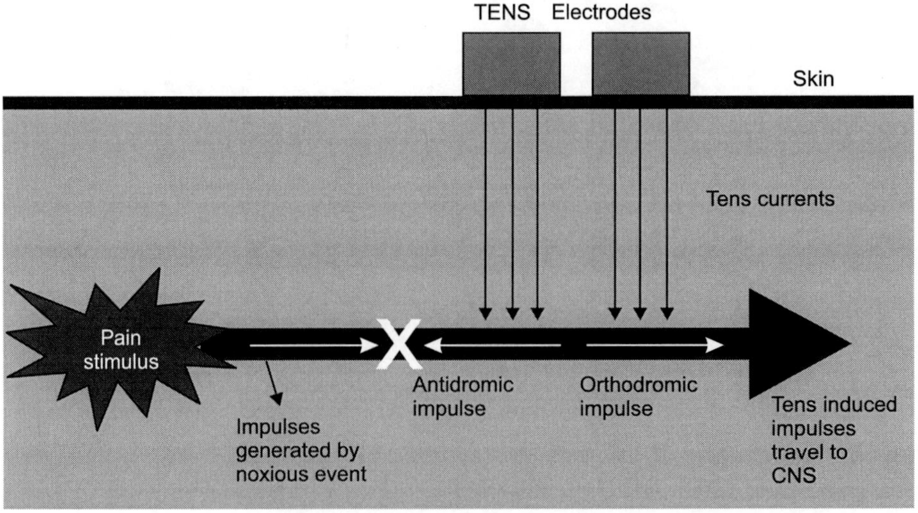

Fig. 48.9: Peripheral mechanism

PRACTICAL APPROACH TO PAIN GATE THEORIES

Before going to practical approach to pain gate theories, it is better to understand the classification of nerve fibers. Table 48.5 shows the classification of nerve fibers according to the velocity, function, frequency and its physiological blocking. Frequency means to stimulate a particular nerve fibers and blocking means frequency to stop conducting impulse in a nerve fiber. NA means not applicable.

Table 48.5: Classification of nerve fibers with its velocity, frequency and blocking

Nerve fiber	*Function*	*Velocity*	*Frequency*	*Blocking*
A alpha, Ia	Motor efferent Muscle spindle afferent	120–70	10–50	>50 tetanic
A beta, II	Mechano receptors	70–30	80–100	>135
A gamma	Intrafusal	30–15	NA	NA
A delta	Fast pain	30–12	25–40	>40
B	Pre–ganglionic	10–3	1–10	>15
C	Post–ganglionic Chronic pain	2–0.5	10–15	>15

Relief of Acute Pain

Acute pain can be relieved by either stimulating A–beta (A-β) fibers or block A–delta (A-δ) fibers. From the Table 48.5, it is understood that the optimal firing rate to stimulate A-β fibers is by keeping in between 80 and 100 Hz and to block A-δ should be kept above 40 Hz (Fig. 48.10).

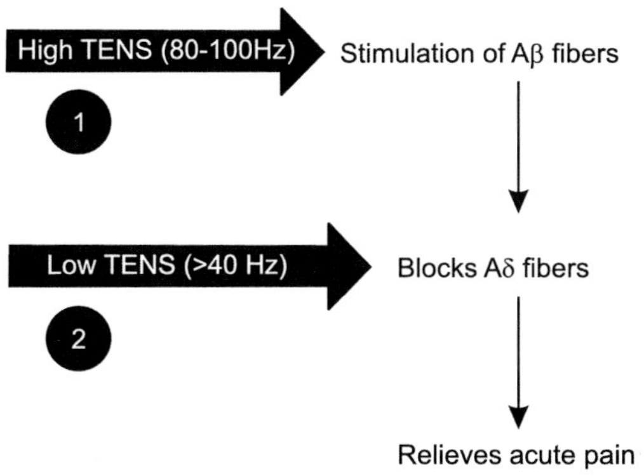

Fig. 48.10: Mechanism of acute pain relief

Relief of Chronic Pain

Chronic pain can be relieved by either stimulating A–Alpha (A-α) fibers, A–delta (A-δ) fibers, C fibers or blocking C fibers. From the Table 48.5, it is understood that a therapist can choose any of the following four options as mentioned below for firing or block an optimal fiber (Fig. 48.11).

1. Stimulating A–alpha (A-α) fibers: By keeping in between 1 and 10 Hz.

   Stimulation of A–alpha fibers results in a muscle twitch in a painful area. This results in acute pain. This is carried by A–delta (A-δ) fibers which blocks C fiber transmission at spinal cord level, thereby relieving chronic pain.
2. Stimulating A–delta (A-δ) fibers: By keeping in between 25 and 40 Hz.
3. Blocking C fibers: By keeping above 15 Hz.
4. Stimulating C fibers: By keeping in between 10 and 15 Hz.

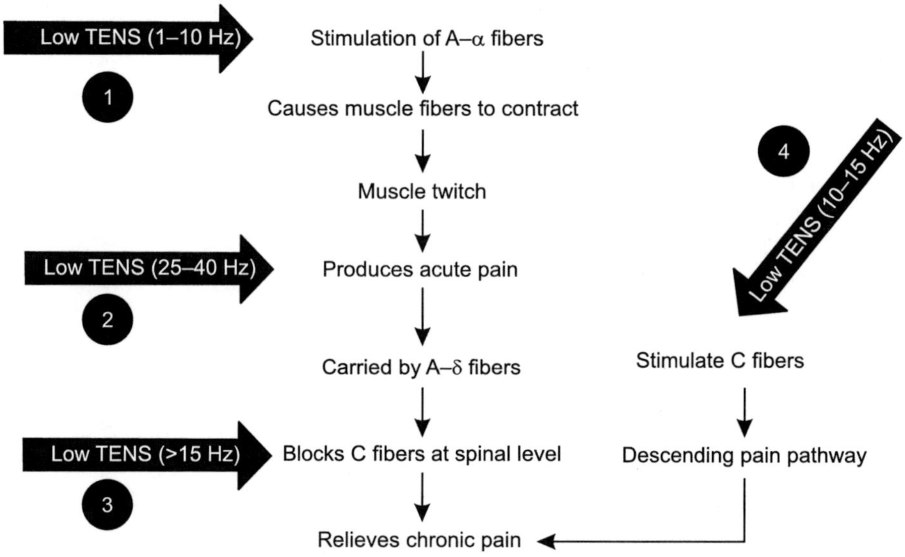

Fig. 48.11: Mechanism of chronic pain relief

Relief of Numbness

As numbness is carried by A-beta fibers, it can be blocked by keeping above 135 Hz with high intensity.

Limitations of Gate Control Theory

(i) It does not clarify the role of afferent synapses in lamina I although they have been shown to be receptive to noxious stimuli.

(ii) It does not account for peripheral blocking mechanism.

(iii) It does not explain why patients with poly neuropathies that destroy large fibers do not have pain.

(iv) It does not explain why thallium induced poly neuropathy continue to experience pain although they should not.

49

TENS

DEFINITION

TENS is the application of low frequency current through the surface electrode on the patient's skin to reduce the pain.

CHARACTERISTICS

- Pulse waveform: Monophasic or Biphasic symmetrical or Biphasic asymmetrical and balanced
- Pulse shape: Rectangular
- Pulse amplitude: 0–60 milli ampere
- Pulse duration : 10–1000 micro second
- Pulse frequency: 1–200 Hz
- It can be battery operated or through AC operated.

TYPES (Fig. 49.1)

1. High TENS (Conventional TENS)

This type of application is high frequency low intensity TENS. It is used for relief of acute pain. The mechanism is blocking Aδ by stimulating Aβ fibers. Treatment has to be given for a minimum period of 40 minutes to one hour. By the applications of TENS, patient feels a soothing effect immediately. This effect is continued till the treatment is given. There is no carry over effect (the effect is lost when the treatment is stopped).

2. Low TENS (Acupuncture TENS)

This type of application is low frequency high intensity TENS. It is mainly used for relief of chronic pain. This application is painful to the patient. Low TENS stimulate A α fibers (1–10 Hz) which causes muscle contraction. Muscle twitch in a painful site produces an acute pain. This sensation is carried by Aδ fibers which block C fibers at spinal cord level. Another mechanism of pain relief is by directly stimulating Aδ by keeping 25–40 Hz which blocks C – fibers or by keeping 10–15 Hz which stimulates C fibers which goes through descending pathway which blocks C fibers transmission. Treatment time of low TENS application is generally for 20 minutes. There is no immediate effect with this technique and no effect during the treatment session. But, there is a carryover effect which last longer.

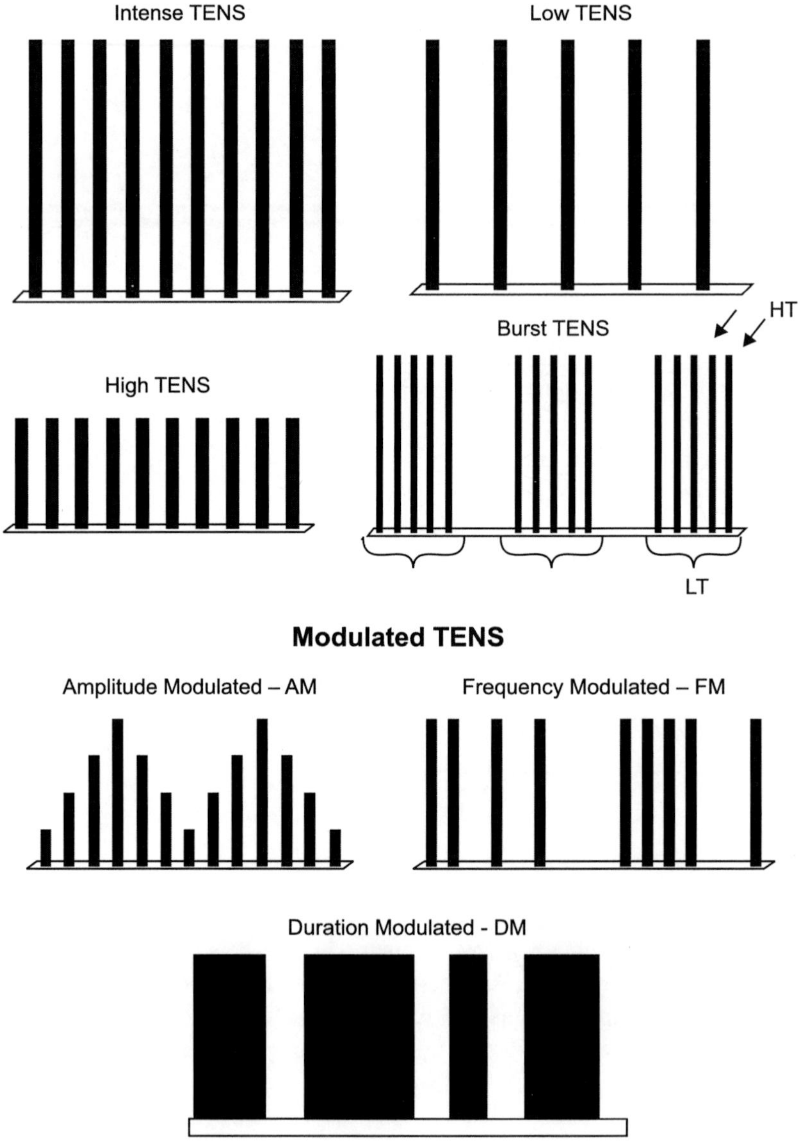

Fig. 49.1: Types of TENS

3. Intense TENS (Brief TENS)

This type of application is high frequency high intensity TENS. It is commonly used for relief of postoperative pain. The mechanism of pain relief is by peripheral mechanism (already explained in the previous chapter). Application of intense TENS results in activation of Aδ fibers. There will be peripheral blockage of nociceptor afferent (by blocking the orthodromic transmissions by antidromic conduction of TENS application. Brain perceives pain due to the TENS stimulation not from the painful site. Treatment time administered is usually less than 5 minutes.

4. Dual TENS

In the dual TENS application, two channels from a single machine is delivered. It can be used to treat two patient at a time, can treat two different side of the same patient, can treat using both the channel in same patient if the area to be treated is large, can treat same patient at same site using high TENS at both channels or low TENS at both channels or one high and other low. Dual TENS is also used to treat multiple joints

5. Burst TENS

A series of burst of pulses is administered. Each pulse within the burst will act as a high TENS while each burst will act as a low TENS. This can be used for the relief of acute pain and chronic pain at the same site. A condition like acute on chronic is most suited for this application. For example, patient is diagnosed with back pain for long period (chronic) suddenly pain was increased from two days (acute).

6. Modulated TENS

Nerve get adapted with TENS application so the intensity has to be increased periodically to prevent it. This nerve habituation can be prevented with the application of modulated TENS. In modulated TENS frequency, duration and amplitude automatically varies during the progression of treatment session.

Comparison of high TENS, low TENS and Intense TENS is detailed in Table 49.1.

PHYSIOLOGICAL EFFECTS OF TENS

1. **Analgesic effect**
   Works on the principles of pain gate theory
   - Segmental mechanism
   - Extra-segmental mechanism
   - Descending pathway
   - Peripheral mechanism
2. **Non-analgesic effect**
   - Antiemetic effect: It reduces vomiting sensation or nausea in pregnant ladies.
   - Restoration of blood flow: Dilation of blood vessels due to stimulation.

Table 49.1: Comparison of conventional, Acupuncture and intense TENS

Sl. No.	*Features*	*Conventional TENS*	*Acupuncture TENS*	*Intense TENS*
1	Synonym	High TENS	Low TENS	Brief TENS
2	Frequency	High frequency low intensity	Low frequency High intensity	High frequency High intensity
3	Mechanism of action	Stimulate Aβ, blocks Aδ (relief of Acute pain)	1. Stimulate Aα fiber; Muscle contracts; cause acute pain; carried by Aδ and blocks C fiber 2. Stimulate directly Aδ which blocks C fibers 3. Stimulating C fibers blocking the same C fibers 4. Block C fibers	Blocking the orthodromic transmissions by antidromic conduction of TENS application
4	Mechanism of pain relief	Segmental mechanism	Extra segmental mechanism Descending pain pathway	Peripheral mechanism
5	Patient experience	Strong sensory stimulation pin prickling sensation without muscle contraction (ant crawling sensation)	Intensity will be high and painful muscle contraction	Intensity should be high. Pain and muscle contraction should be minimal
6	Position of the electrode	Cathode proximal, anode distal	Anode proximal, cathode distal	Either both the electrode proximal to the incision or on the either side of incision
7	Placement of electrode	Over the dermatome	Over the myotome, motor point, trigger point	Proximal to the site of incision or adjacent
8	Characteristics or the effects	Rapid onset Rapid offset	Delayed onset Delayed offset	Rapid onset Delayed offset
9	Duration of the treatment	Minimum 45 minutes ideally up to one hour	10-20 minutes	Less than 5 minutes
10	Pulse characteristics (a) Frequency	80–100 Hz	1–5 Hz	100–150 Hz
	(b) Pulse width	100–500 microsec	100–150 microsec	100–500 microsec
	(c) Amplitude/Intensity	12–30 mA	Greater than 30 mA	Greater than 30 mA
11	Pain relief	Relief of acute pain	Relief of chronic pain	Relief of postoperative pain

THERAPEUTIC EFFECTS

1. Relief of acute pain
2. Relief of chronic pain
3. Antiemetic effect
4. Relief of nausea
5. Improved blood flow
6. Reduction of ischemia
7. Increased healing/improve healing of wound

Relief of Acute Pain (Fig. 48.10)

Acute pain can be relieved by either stimulating A–beta (A-β) fibers or block A–delta (A-δ) fibers. From the Table 48.5 it is understood that the optimal firing rate to stimulate A-β fibers is by keeping in between 80 and 100 Hz and to block A-δ should be kept above 40 Hz.

Relief of Chronic Pain (Fig. 48.11)

Chronic pain can be relieved by either stimulating A–alpha (A-α) fibers, A–delta (A-δ) fibers, C fibers or blocking C fibers. A therapist can choose any of the following four options as mentioned below for fire or block an optimal fiber.

1. Stimulating A–alpha (A-α) fibers: By keeping in between 1–10 Hz.

Stimulation of A–alpha fibers results in a muscle twitch in a painful area. This results in acute pain. This is carried by A–delta (A-δ) fibers which blocks C fiber transmission at spinal cord level, thereby relieving chronic pain.

2. Stimulating A-delta (A-δ) fibers: By keeping in between 25 and 40 Hz.
3. Blocking C fibers: By keeping above 15 Hz.
4. Stimulating C fibers: By keeping in between 10 and 15 Hz.

INDICATIONS

1. Acute pain:
   (a) Low back pain
   (b) Postoperative pain (both thoracic or abdominal)
   (c) Labor and post–labor pain
   (d) Painful menstruation
   (e) Musculoskeletal pain
   (f) During dental procedures.
2. Relief of chronic pain:
   (a) Low back pain
   (b) Neck pain
   (c) Radiating pain
   (d) All type of arthritis (juvenile, osteo, Rheumatoid)
   (e) Stump or phantom limb pain.
3. Other types:
   (a) Post hepatic neuralgia
   (b) Causalgia–abnormal sensation perceived in intact skin
   (c) Peripheral nerve disorders
   (d) Facial pain (seen in trigeminal neuralgia)
   (e) Metastasis bone pain (pain due to cancer)

   (f) Orofacial pain
   (g) Migraine/Headache.
4. Antiemetic effect:
   (a) Postoperative nausea
   (b) Nausea associated with opoid drug medication
   (c) Nausea associated with chemotherapy
   (d) Early morning sickness (hyperemesis gravidarum).
5. To improve blood flow in case of Raynaud's disease.
6. In reconstructive surgery.
7. Burning sensation in the feet in case of diabetic neuropathy.
8. Improve the healing rate in case of wounds and ulcers.

ELECTRODE PLACEMENT IN TENS

1. At the site of the pain/painful area method – can give high as well as low TENS.
2. Spinal nerve root method – can give high as well as low TENS.
3. Over the dermatome – both high and low TENS.
4. Myotome – low TENS, cathode distal anode proximal.
5. Sclerotome (area of spinal segment supply the particular bone) – both the TENS is used.
6. Over the motor point – low TENS is given.
7. Over acupuncture point – low TENS is given.
8. Over acupressure point – low TENS is given.
9. Along the course of the peripheral nerve – low TENS is given.
10. Over the site of incision after surgery – intense TENS.
11. Over trigger point – low TENS.
12. Preferred stimulation site by Ohm meter. It is a device which tells us about the skin resistance. Electrode is placed where there is less resistance. Both high and low TENS can be given.
13. Over the unrelated extrasegmental site that may contribute to excitation of supra-segmental and cortical pain inhibitory center.
14. Electro acupuncture.

ELECTRODE USED IN TENS

1. Carbon impregnated rubber electrode.
2. Self adhesive electrode.
3. Karaya gel electrode.
4. Butterfly electrode.

   Coupling media: Rubber electrode with electrode gel.

50

Interferential Therapy

HISTORY

Dr Nemec from Vienna, an Austrian physicist (1950).

Earlier it was called as Nemectodyne therapy.

Hanssurgens add vector component to it.

DEFINITION

Transcutaneous application of alternating medium frequency electrical currents, which are slightly out of phase through the tissues, amplitude modulated at low frequency for therapeutic purposes, such as relief of pain, improve circulation and enhance healing process.

PRINCIPLES OF WAVE INTERFERENCE

- Constructive
- Destructive
- Continuous

Constructive interference: When two sinusoidal waves, i.e., exactly in phase, the waves supplement each other in constructive interference (Fig. 50.1).

Destructive interference: When the two waves are different by 1/2 a wavelength (of any multiple) the result is cancellation of both waves (Fig. 50.2).

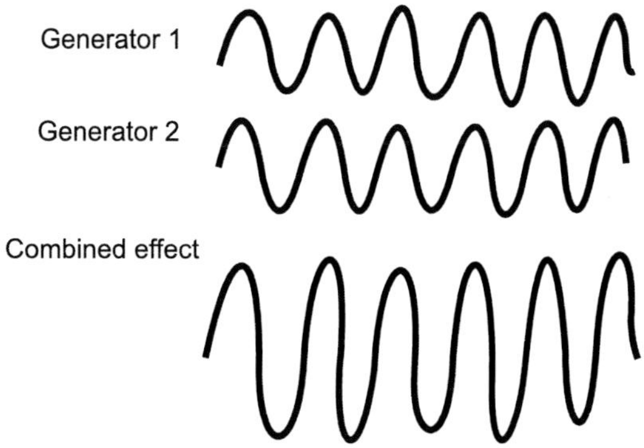

Fig. 50.1: Constructive interference

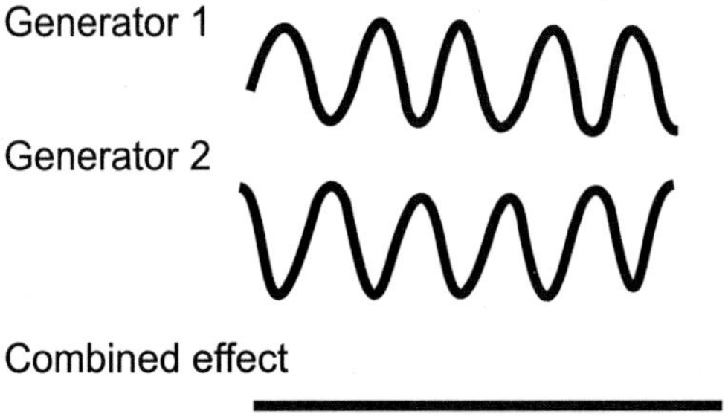

Fig. 50.2: Destructive interference

Continuous Interference: Two waves slightly out of phase collide and form a single wave with progressively increasing and decreasing amplitude (Fig. 50.3).

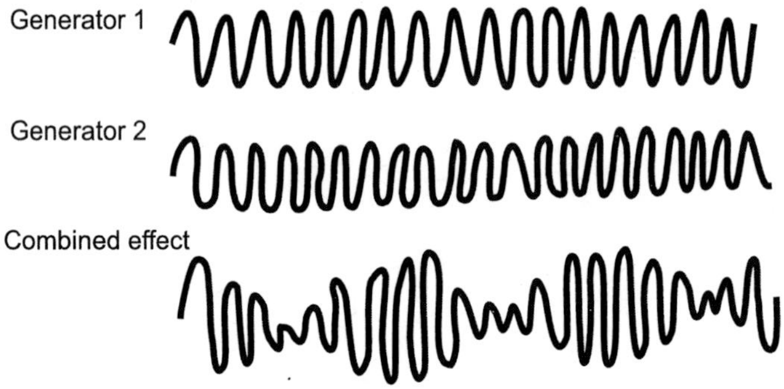

Fig. 50.3: Continuous interference

Thus, Interferential Currents (IFC) are produced. If two generators have slightly different frequencies, they are out of phase and thus, create a *beat* pattern. Blending of waves caused by constructive and destructive interference patterns called *heterodyne* effect. Thus, two medium frequency currents which are applied in a cross pattern a amplitude modulated low frequency is produced at the center (Fig. 50.4).

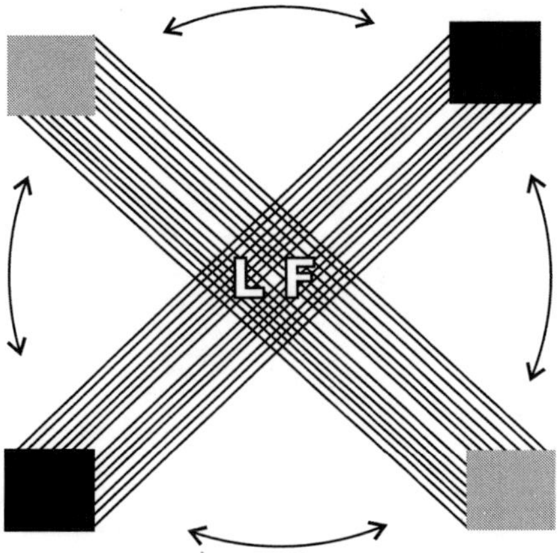

Fig. 50.4: Formation of low frequency current at the center

Amplitude Modulated Frequency (AMF): Defined as the difference between the frequency of two medium frequency currents which is produced in the tissues at the point where two current cross. Amplitude of AMF is always higher than the amplitude of two medium frequency currents. When sine waves from two similar sources have different frequencies are out of phase and blend (heterodyne) to produce the interference beating effect.

Static AMF: By varying frequency of second circuit relative to constant frequency of first, it is possible to produce a range of beat frequency deep in the patient's tissues. It is called as static interference where the area in which IFC is set up remains stationary.

Types

Constant or selective beat frequency: Constant frequency of first and second circuit.

Variable or automatic beat frequency: Constant frequency of first circuit and variable frequency of second circuit.

Purpose of Automatic Beat Frequency

- To prevent nerve habituation
- It can also extend the range of nerve types that can be stimulated.

Dynamic AMF: By incorporating vector in the circuit. Introduction of vector can be produced by continuously changing the amplitude of the circuit one and circuit two. The vector or scanning types are 45° and 90°. This is also called as Dynamic interference where the area in which IFC is developed move in a to and fro manner through 45° or 90°. Advantages are a large area can be treated and there is less need for perfect electrode placement.

Principle of Vector

Assume that F1 is equal to zero then the resultant R will lie along F2 at zero degree. If F2 is equal to zero the resultant R will lie along F1 at 90°. Thus, carrying the intensities of the currents out of phase will shift or the direction of the resulting interference current from zero to 90° (Fig. 50.5).

If no vector is introduced, the field will be limited to area of interference, i.e., area where interferential current is set up. Figure 50.4 in the figure area remains stationary. This area resembles a clover leaf.

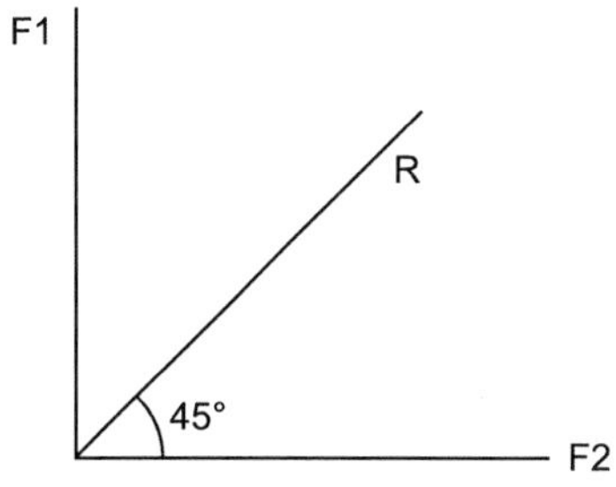

Fig. 50.5: Principle of vector

Clove leaf appearance: Theoretical distribution of current in homogenous medium makes an appearance called clove leaf appearance. Due to the fact that both currents amplitudes and their directions need to be summated, i.e., vector addition. Variation in tissue resistance and electrolyte distance would prevent this appearance. Real pattern is much more irregular and diffuse in all tissues between and around electrodes.

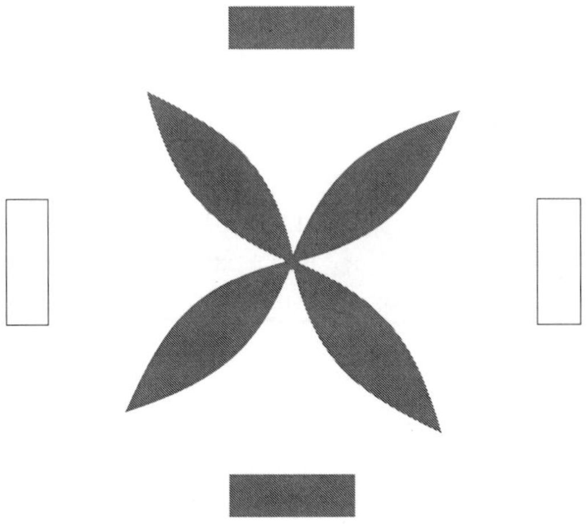

Fig. 50.6: Area of interference without vector

45 degree: By varying the intensity of second circuit relative to the constant intensity of the first (Fig. 50.7). Arrow marked area where the area of interference shifts. It covers small area.

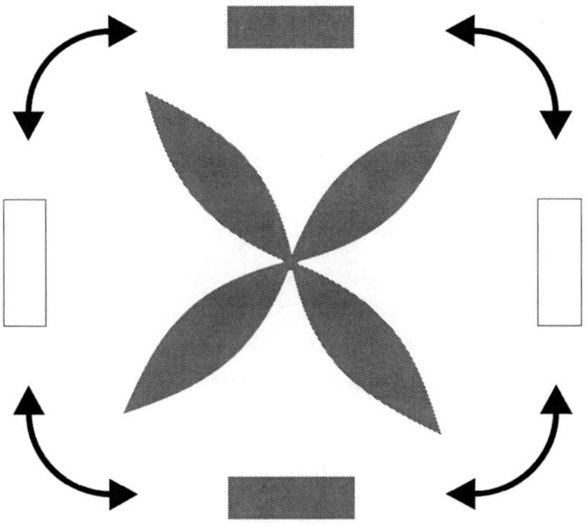

Fig. 50.7: 45 Degree vector

90 degree: Increasing intensity of first while decreasing the intensity of second or vice versa. Current is varied from 50 to 100% (Fig. 50.8). Arrow marked area where the area of interference shifts. It will cover large area.

Purpose:

No vector: if area is too localized.

45 degree: to treat a large area.

90 degree: if area is diffused or cannot be localized.

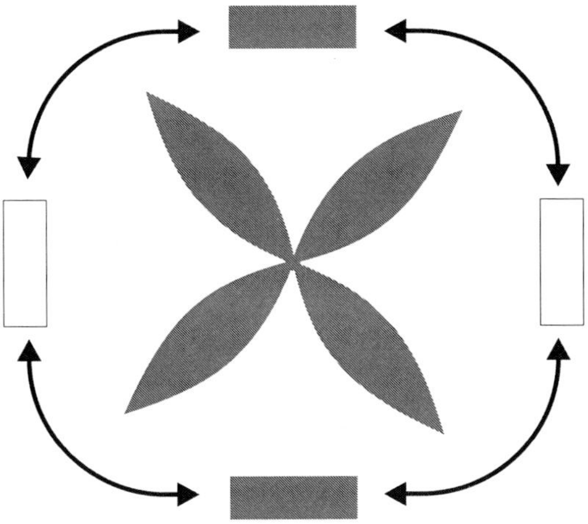

Fig. 50.8: 90 degree vector

PHYSIOLOGICAL AND THERAPEUTIC EFFECTS

1. On Sensory nerves
2. On Motor nerves
3. Decrease pain
4. Decrease edema
5. In tissue healing
6. On involuntary muscles

    1. **On Sensory nerves:** Effect is based on the frequency applied. With low AMF it produces tapping sensation and with high AMF it produces prickling or tingling sensation.
    2. **On motor nerves:** Effect is based on the frequency applied.
        - If it is less than 10 Hz, results in single muscle twitch.
        - If it is between 10–30 Hz, results in summation.
        - If it is more than 50 Hz, results in Tetanic contraction.
    3. **Relief of pain:**
        (a) Segmental mechanism theory 1
        (b) Segmental mechanism theory 2
        (c) Descending pain pathway
        (d) A Physiological block
        (e) Increased circulation
        (f) Placebo effect
        (g) Sympathetic blocking

Description of a, b and c is already given in previous Chapters 47 and 48.

(d) **Physiological blocking:** A physiological blocking is a method by which blocking the transmission of a nerve fiber impulse by keeping frequency above their firing rate. For example, to block A delta fibers keep the frequency above 40 Hz since A–delta fibers conduct the impulse in a range of 25–40 Hz. Blocking frequency of nerve fibers are mentioned below:

A–beta > 135 Hz

A–delta > 40 Hz

C fibers > 15 Hz.

(e) **Increased circulation:** Increased circulation results in removal of substance which stimulates pain nerve ending from within the damaged area.

(f) **Placebo effect:** Placebo is defined as a positive or negative response to a therapy resulting from person's expectations rather than from any real effects. IFT is bigger equipment so it is impressive. Color of electrodes, flashing lights and noises produces overall a placebo effect.

(g) **Sympathetic blocking:** Mascular coat of small arterioles of body is innervated by sympathetic fibers. A depressive effect on this system is intended to produce an increased blood flow through the part, hence removing the pain producing substances. Additional blood flowing though the part removes the edematous fluid away from it. As a result, it removes waste product and bring nutrients for healing.

4. **Control and Reduction of Edema:**

- Sensory Level (acute edema): Limit edema formation before it appears.
- Motor Level (chronic edema): Remove existing edema.

Acute edema

With IFC there is oscillation of more marked amplitude than short waves which is at much higher frequency. There will be rapid fine vibrations of ions without heat. There will be alteration in caliber of vessels which reduces micro vessel diameter. This further reduces microvessel permeability. As a normal response to trauma, there is production of histamine. As a result pores would be enlarged. With IFC there is reduction in pore size in microvessel wall thereby preventing large plasma protein leaking through pores. There will be also the repolarization of already depolarized membranes due to trauma.

5. **Role of tissue healing:**

Already described in the previous Chapter 32.

6. **Action on involuntary visceral muscle:** Effect is either directly or through autonomic mechanisms. Zero to ten frequencies used for atonic colons and for weak sphincters. 100 Hz is used to relax spastic colon.

IFT PARAMETERS

Frequency Knob: Either 2 KHz or 4 KHz.

2 KHz is preferred for motor stimulation and 4 KHz is preferred for pain relief. As 2 KHz is not tolerated by elderly for muscle stimulation, 4 KHz is given for the same.

Frequency Sweep: It can be Triangular, Rectangular or Trapezoidal.

***Triangular sweep*:** The machine gradually changes from the base to the top frequency, usually over a time period of 6 seconds – though some machines offer 1 or 3 second options. In the example illustrated (Fig. 50.9), the machine is set to sweep from 80 to 100 Hz employing a triangular sweep pattern. All frequencies between the base and top frequencies are delivered in equal proportion.

So, a triangular sweep is used to prevent nerve habituation or it is used to stimulate one nerve at a time.

In the above example, A triangular sweep will stimulate A–beta nerve without getting habituated.

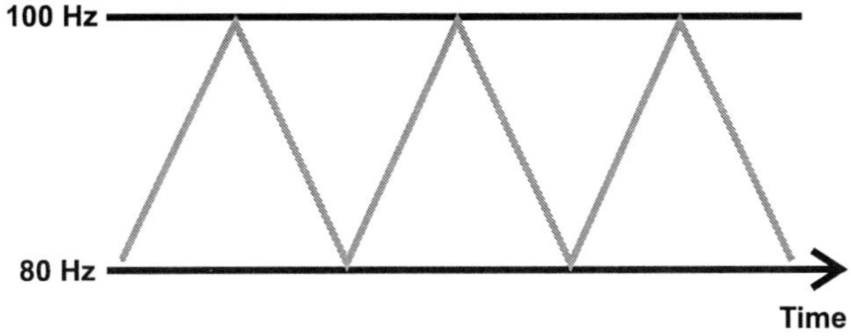

Fig. 50.9: Triangular sweep

***Rectangular sweep*:** This produces a very different stimulation pattern in that the base and top frequencies are set, but the machine then 'switches' between these two specific frequencies rather than gradually changing from one to the other. Figure 50.10 illustrates the effect of setting a 40–90 Hz rectangular sweep. **It is used to stimulate two nerves at a time.**

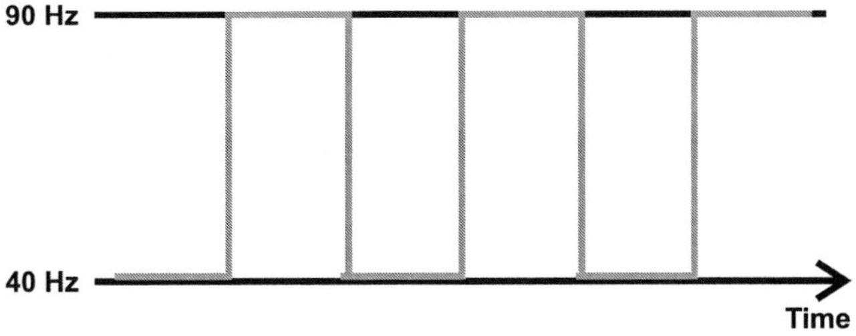

Fig. 50.10: Rectangular sweep

In the above example, setting at lower frequency 40 Hz will block A delta fibers and setting a 90 Hz will stimulate A beta which further blocks A delta sensations. Both relieves acute pain.

Trapezoidal: There is a clear difference between triangular and trapezoidal. Even though the same 'numbers' are set. One will deliver a full range of stimulation frequencies between the set frequency levels and the other will switch from one frequency to the other. So, a trapezoidal pulse can effectively stimulate one nerve fiber at base, one at between base and spectrum and the third one at spectrum. **So it is used to stimulate three nerves at a time.** In the given example (Fig. 50.11), if we want to relieve chronic pain by inhibiting C fibers, stimulating A–delta fibers and A–alpha fibers trapezoidal sweep is the optimum choice.

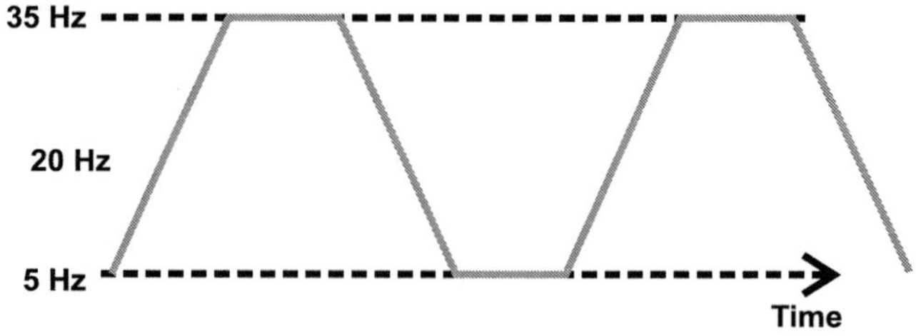

Fig. 50.11: Trapezoidal sweep

Base, Sweep, Spectrum

Care needs to be taken when setting the sweep on a machine in that with some devices, the user sets the actual base and top frequencies (e.g., 10 and 25 Hz) and with other machines the user sets the base frequency and then how much needs to be added for the fluctuated (e.g., 10 and 15 Hz). So, spectrum is the top frequency and how much fluctuation added is sweep.

Current Intensity

Less than 8 mA is preferred for sensory stimulation and more than 8 mA for motor stimulation. Patient should feel 'Strong but comfortable' sensation. It should be subject report rather than current settings. Sensation varies between individual and over time, area treated and size and placement of electrodes.

Balance

Purpose of balance is to produce equal sensation under four electrodes. Since two circuits are present and if one circuit slightly longer than other pathway then the intensity must be adjusted to meet this difference. If it is not used, select the knob to midline. Control can be rotated by a small margin on either side of center line.

METHODS OF APPLICATION

It can be quadripolar with four electrodes or bipolar with two electrodes. The details are mentioned in the Table 50.1.

Table 50.1: Method of application

Quadripolar application	*Bipolar application*
Applying the two medium frequency currents via four electrodes so that they intersect in the tissues	Alternatively by mixing the two currents in the stimulator prior to application via two electrodes premodulated
Endogenously in the tissues	Exogenously outside the tissues
Used to treat larger areas	Used to treat smaller areas
Modulation in the form of Clove leaf pattern	100% modulation under the electrodes

TYPES OF ELECTRODES

Electrodes used in IFT can be rubber electrodes, suction electrodes (vacuum electrode) or combined electrodes.

Carbon or rubber electrodes are easier to apply on peripheral limbs with bandages and Velcro straps. They are described in the Chapter 30. Compared to NMES larger electrodes are preferred. In this method, coupling media is generally Spontex material which is soaked in water or a solution of soda bicarbonate to improve conduction. This allows comfortable contact with skin. In order to prevent cross infection, it has to be washed thoroughly in disinfectant. The rubber electrodes are attached to the patient (binding) by means of straps or crepe bandages. Straps can be applied quickly and easily but the crepe bandage gives a firmer and even contact which results in a comfortable treatment. In vacuum electrodes, the plates are kept in position by vacuum instead of bandaging.

Vacuum Electrode (Suction electrode) is administered to the patients who are relatively immobile, to the areas less accessible. Vacuum electrode is a type of electrode which is like a rubber cap. Here, the electrode is kept at the base of rubber cap and wire or lead is connected at narrow end. Generally, a soaked sponge or spontex is kept just below the electrode so as to achieve even contact to skin and hence, better conduction. Round edge of the cup is flange to allow airtight seal which is made with the patient's skin. These electrodes are held in position with negative pressure created by a vacuum pump. It produces vacuum effect thereby stimulating cutaneous nerves and causes vasodilatation. The magnitude of the vacuum should be adjusted so that the least amount of suction is necessary to keep the electrodes on the skin otherwise superficial bruising may occur. If the electrodes are removed without the release of vacuum results in discomfort and bruising. Vacuum electrodes are excellent for treating flat smooth areas, such as the back or knee. It is difficult to hold vacuum electrodes on bony areas, such as shoulder and ankle.

Contraindication to vacuum electrodes:

- Hemorrhage or bruising is present.
- On hairy areas: difficult to get air tight seal.
- Elderly: as skin is thin, this may result in bruises.
- Patients on steroid therapy: results in bruising.

Combined electrodes are constructed such a way that all four contacts are embedded in some insulating materials and can be applied as one pad. They are made up of small, medium and large sizes. In the smallest size all electrodes are enclosed in 2.5 cm in diameter. The effect is very superficial. This electrode is mainly used to treat small nerve arises from the foramen. The medium sized electrode has four contacts, each 1 cm in diameter. This is used to treat finger joints. The largest size has contacts about 5 cm across. It is used for the treatment of wrist or elbow in a thin patient.

Labile electrode is a plate electrode insulated on one side and attached to the operators hand by means of Velcro straps. The conducting side is covered with Spontex to provide contact. Two electrodes are used. They are held in position by the therapist and designed to be moved over the patient's skin during treatment.

ELECTRODE PLACEMENT IN IFT

Either painful area method or spinal nerve root placement is preferred for nonradiating back or neck pain (Already mentioned in the previous chapter). Electrodes are placed along the nerve root in case of radiating pain.

ADVANTAGES

- Less sensory nerve irritation
- Deep
- Localized versus extensive area
- Less skin resistance
- Metals not contraindicated
- No fatigue
- Acute case – no heat is produced
- Rapid return of tone of pelvic floor
- Patient can move while having treatment
- It is not necessary to have intact sensation
- Long lasting effect.

DISADVANTAGES

- Unable to voluntarily contract with current
- Expensive and bulky
- Not portable
- Eliminates pain but do not treat cause of pain, may mask serious problem
- Supervision of therapist is required.

INDICATIONS

Same as that of TENS for all types of pain relief

In women's health: Conditions, like Stress incontinence, Dysmenorrhea, Uterovaginal prolapse, etc.

Vascular disease: Sudecks atrophy, Raynaud's disease.

Sports injuries.

Contraindications dangers and precautions are covered in Chapter 37.

SPECIAL PRECAUTIONS

When treating transthoracic area intensity should be less than 60 mA or else results in ventricular fibrillation.

Hot Spot

WEDINSKY INHIBITION

Loss of excitation caused by maintaining a continuous refractory state with constant amplitude stimulus of frequency greater than 1000 Hz is called wedinsky inhibition.

GLIDEMEISTER EFFECT

With medium frequency biphasic pulses, the depolarization frequency of nerve fibers coincides neither with frequency of current nor with depolarization frequency of other nerve fibers in the nerve bundle. Summation of several cycles of biphasic pulses is needed to depolarize even the lowest threshold nerve fibers.

Appendix

SETTING THE BASE, SWEEP AND SPECTRUM IN INTERFERENTIAL THERAPY

While setting IFT parameters, Physiotherapist always get confused with setting the base and spectrum. Because of this, Physiotherapist treats the patient with programmed mode in IFT. A manual mode technique is better than a programmed mode, if applied properly. Before going into this topic I would ask the readers to go through the pain gate theories, mechanism of relieving acute and chronic pain, basics of IFT from the previous chapters of this book.

Relief of Acute Pain

Acute pain can be relieved by either stimulating A beta (A-β) fibers or block A delta (A-δ) fibers. The optimal firing rate to stimulate A-β fibers is by keeping in between 80 and 100 Hz and to block A-δ should be kept above 40 Hz.

Relief of Chronic Pain

Chronic pain can be relieved by either stimulating A Alpha (A-α) fibers, A delta (A-δ) fibers, C fibers or blocking C fibers. A therapist can choose any of the following four options as mentioned below for stimulate or inhibit nerve fiber.

- Stimulation of A alpha (A-α) fibers results in a muscle twitch in a painful area. This results in acute pain. This is carried by A delta (A-δ) fibers which blocks C fiber transmission at spinal cord level, thereby relieving chronic pain.
- Stimulating A delta (A-δ) fibers: By keeping in between 25 and 40 Hz.
- Stimulating C fibers: By keeping in between 10 and 15 Hz.
- Blocking C fibers: By keeping above 15 Hz (this option should be used in TENS, not in IFT).

Base, Sweep and Spectrum

Base is the lowest frequency to set, spectrum is the top frequency and how much fluctuation added is sweep.

In simple words

Base + sweep = spectrum

Setting Base and Spectrum in Acute Pain

The optimal firing rate to stimulate A-β fibers is by keeping in between 80 and 100 Hz. In this case base is 80 and spectrum is 100. In some machine instead of spectrum, sweep frequency is present. So to set sweep subtract base from spectrum that is 20 in this example. When only one nerve fiber is targeted always a triangular sweep waveform is selected.

In triangular sweep all frequencies between the base and top frequencies are delivered in equal proportion. Acute pain also can be relieved by inhibiting A delta fibers. In this case base will be 41and spectrum will be below 79 (A delta stimulating frequency is between 25 and 40). Hence the base is above this. Since the next nerve fiber; A beta stimulating range is 80-100 Hz, the spectrum should be kept below 80 Hz.

In summary for a triangular mode either of the following options is used:

(1) Base: above 81, spectrum below 99.

(2) Base: 41, spectrum below 79.

A rectangular sweep is used if u wants to stimulate two nerve fibers at a time. So for relieving acute pain either stimulate A beta (between 80 and 100) or inhibit A delta (between 41 and 60). In this case base can be kept as 41 and spectrum as 100 (here the four frequency numbers are 80, 100, 41 and 60. Arrange it in ascending order. The lowest will be base and highest will be spectrum.

Setting Base and Spectrum in Chronic Pain

Chronic pain can be relieved by three mechanisms either stimulate A alpha or stimulate A delta or inhibit C fibers. A triangular sweep mode is used for stimulating any one nerve at a time. Stimulate A alpha (base 1 spectrum 9), stimulate A delta (base 26 spectrum 39), inhibit C fibers (base 16 spectrum 24). A rectangular sweep is used for stimulating two nerves at a time.

Any of the three following combinations can be used:

Stimulate A alpha and stimulate A delta: Base will be 1 spectrum will be 39 (Arrange frequencies in ascending order). The lowest will be base and highest will be spectrum.

- Stimulate A alpha and inhibit C fibers: Base will be 1 spectrum will be 24.
- Stimulate A delta and inhibit C fibers: Base will be 16 and spectrum will be 39.

A trapezoidal sweep will be used to stimulate three nerves at a time.

Stimulate A alpha, stimulate A delta or inhibit C fibers. (Here the frequency 1-10, 26-39, 15-24. Arrange it in ascending order lowest is base: 1 and highest is spectrum: 39).

REFERENCES

1. Alex R Ward. *Biophysical basis of electrotherapy.* Available online at http://www.docfoc.com/alex-ward-biophysical-bases-of-electrotherapy.
2. Angela Forster and Nigel Palastanga. *Clayton's Electrotherapy: Theory and Practice:* 9th edn. (Physiotherapy Essentials) 1985.
3. Anilkumar J. Shinde, Amit L. Shinde, Kevin C. Garala, Sachin A. Kandekar, Harinath N. More. *Physical Penetration Enhancement By Iontophoresis: A Review International Journal of Current Pharmaceutical Research* 2010;2(1): 1–9.
4. Ashish Kakkad. *Fundamentals of Electrotherapy and Biomedical Physics*. Jaypee Brothers Medical Publishers, 1st edn., 2014. Print.
5. Bélanger A. *Therapeutic Electrophysical Agents*. Philadelphia: Wolters Kluwer Health/Lippincott Williams and Wilkins, 2010.
6. Cameron, Michelle H. *Physical Agents in Rehabilitation.* St Louis, Mo.: Saunders/Elsevier, 2009. Print.
7. Clayton, E. Bellis, Angela Forster, Nigel Palastanga. *Clayton's Electrotherapy*. London: Baillière Tindall, 1985. Print.
8. Fox, John, Tim Sharp, Sheila Kitchen. *Practical Electrotherapy*. Edinburgh: Churchill Livingstone, 2007. Print.
9. Gersh, Meryl R. *Electrotherapy in Rehabilitation*. Philadelphia: Davis, 1992. Print.
10. Jagmohan Singh. *Textbook of Electrotherapy*. New Delhi: Jaypee Brothers Medical Publishers, 2012. Print.
11. Singh, Jagmohan. *Manual of Practical Electrotherapy*. New Delhi: Jaypee Brothers Medical Publishers 2011. Print.
12. John Low, Ann Reed. *Electrotherapy Explained: Principles and Practice*. Butterworth Heineman; 2nd edn. 1995.
13. John Low, Ann Reed. *Electrotherapy Explained: Principles and Practice*. Butterworth Heineman; 3rd edn., 1999.
14. Kitchen Sheila. *Electrotherapy Evidenced Based Practice*, 11th edn., Melbourne/India Elsevier, 2006. Print.
15. Kitchen Sheila, Sarah Bazin, E Bellis Clayton. *Clayton's Electrotherapy*. London: Saunders, 1996. Print.
16. Linda C. Li, Roger A. Scudds. *Iontophoresis: An Overview of the Mechanisms and Clinical Application American College of Rheumatology* 1995;8(1):51–61.
17. Low John, Ann Reed. *Physical Principles Explained*. Oxford: Butterworth-Heinemann, 1994. Print.
18. Nanda Basanta Kumar. *Electrotherapy Simplified*. New Delhi: Jaypee Brothers Medical Publishers 2008. Print.
19. Nelson Roger M, Karen W Hayes, Dean P Currier. *Clinical Electrotherapy*. Stamford, Conn.: Appleton and Lange, 1999. Print.
20. Pauline M. Scott. *Clayton's Electrotherapy and Actinotherapy. A textbook for student physiotherapists.* Bailliere Tindall and Cassell Publishers, 4th Edn., 1962.
21. Petr Slovak, Matej Slovak, Dr. C. Tucker *"Welcome/REBOX THERAPY", 2016. Reboxtherapy.Eu. http://www.reboxtherapy.eu.*
22. Prentice William E and William E Prentice. *Therapeutic Modalities for Physical Therapists.* New York: McGraw-Hill, 2002. Print.
23. Prentice William E, *et al. Therapeutic Modalities in Rehabilitation.* New York: McGraw-Hill, Medical Pub. Division, 2005. Print.
24. Pushpal Kumar Mitra. *Hand Book of Practical Electrotherapy*. Jaypee Brothers Medical Publishers; 1st edn., 2007. Print.
25. Robertson VJ, John Low. *Electrotherapy Explained*. Edinburgh: Butterworth-Heinemann Elsevier, 4th edn.,2006. Print.
26. Robinson Andrew J; Lynn Snyder-Mackler. *Clinical Electrophysiology*. Philadelphia: Wolters Kluwer Health/ Lippincott Williams and Wilkins, 2008. Print.
27. Subash Katri. *Basics of Electrotherapy*. Jaypee Brothers Medical Publishers; 2nd edn., 2012. Print.
28. Sussman Carrie, Barbara M Bates-Jensen. *Wound Care.* Philadelphia: Wolters Kluwer Health/Lippincott Williams and Wilkins, 2012. Print.
29. Tim Watson, Prof. 2016. *"Electrotherapy on the Web". Electrotherapy.Org. http://www.electrotherapy.org/.*
30. Wadsworth, Hilary, APP Chanmugam. *Electrophysical Agents in Physiotherapy.* Marrickville, NSW: Science Press, 1983. Print.
31. Watson, Tim. *Electrotherapy.* Edinburgh: Churchill Livingstone, 2008. Print.
32. *https://www.researchgate.net/publication/345758148_SETTING_THE_BASE_SWEEP_AND_SPECTRUM_IN_INTERFERENTIAL_THERAPY*

    also watch practical approach to pain gate theories animated created at You tube, URLis https://www.youtube.com/watch?v=V8RelKKjPF8.